Medical Billing and Coding
DeMYSTiFieD

Notice

Medicine is an ever-changing science. As new research and clinical experience broaden our knowledge, changes in treatment and drug therapy are required. The authors and the publisher of this work have checked with sources believed to be reliable in their efforts to provide information that is complete and generally in accord with the standards accepted at the time of publication. However, in view of the possibility of human error or changes in medical sciences, neither the authors nor the publisher nor any other party who has been involved in the preparation or publication of this work warrants that the information contained herein is in every respect accurate or complete, and they disclaim all responsibility for any errors or omissions or for the results obtained from use of the information contained in this work. Readers are encouraged to confirm the information contained herein with other sources. For example and in particular, readers are advised to check the product information sheet included in the package of each drug they plan to administer to be certain that the information contained in this work is accurate and that changes have not been made in the recommended dose or in the contraindications for administration. This recommendation is of particular importance in connection with new or infrequently used drugs.

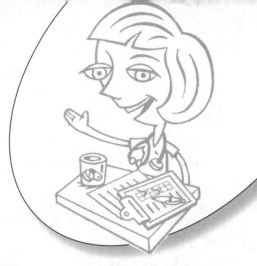

Medical Billing and Coding

DeMYSTiFieD

Second Edition

Marilyn Burgos, BSBA
Donya P. Johnson, BS
Jim Keogh RN-BC, MSN

With contributions by Marissa Hernandez

New York   Chicago   San Francisco   Athens   London   Madrid
Mexico City   Milan   New Delhi   Singapore   Sydney   Toronto

Medical Billing and Coding Demystified, Second Edition

1 2 3 4 5 6 7 8 9 0   DOC/DOC   20 19 18 17 16 15

ISBN   978-0-07-184934-0
MHID   0-07-184934-3

This book was set in Minion Pro by Cenveo® Publisher Services.
The editors were Andrew Moyer and Cindy Yoo.
The production supervisor was Richard Ruzycka.
Project management was provided by Tanya Punj, Cenveo Publisher Services.
RR Donnelley was printer and binder.

This book is printed on acid-free paper.

Library of Congress Cataloging-in-Publication Data

Burgos, Marilyn, author.
    Medical billing and coding demystified / Marilyn Burgos, Donya Johnson, Jim Keogh.—Second edition.
        p. ; cm.—(Demystified series)
    Includes index.
    ISBN 978-0-07-184934-0 (pbk. : alk. paper)—ISBN 0-07-184934-3 (pbk. : alk. paper)
    I. Johnson, Donya, author.   II. Keogh, James Edward, 1948-, author.   III. Title.
    IV. Series: McGraw-Hill "Demystified" series.
    [DNLM: 1. Practice Management—economics—Handbooks.   2. Clinical Coding—Handbooks.
    3. Patient Credit and Collection—Handbooks.   4. Reimbursement Mechanisms—Handbooks.   W 49]
    R728.5
    651.5'04261—dc23

                                                                                    2015026321

McGraw-Hill Education books are available at special quantity discounts to use as premiums and sales promotions or for use in corporate training programs. To contact a representative, please visit the Contact Us pages at www.mhprofessional.com.

I want to thank God for allowing me the privilege and opportunity to be a coauthor for this book. Thank you Jim for working diligently and patiently with us—it has been a wonderful experience. To all my mentors in the medical field, thank you for your insight, support, and guidance which has helped shape me into the healthcare professional I am today. For my beautiful daughter Emilie Rose, who has always been my enthusiastic supporter; may you grow up and stay as enthusiastic in all that you set your mind to. Those who say it cannot be done should not interrupt the person doing it.

—Marilyn Burgos, BSBA

I would have fainted had I failed to see the goodness of God.
Thank You Glenn, Dianne, and Jonathan for all of your love and support.

—Donya P. Johnson, BS

This book is dedicated to Anne, Sandy, Joanne, Amber-Leigh Christine, Shawn, Eric, and Amy. Without their help and support, this book couldn't have been written.

—Jim Keogh, RN-BC, MSN

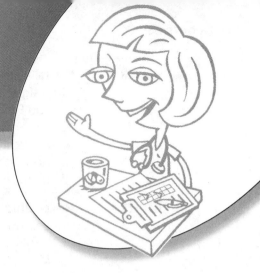

Contents

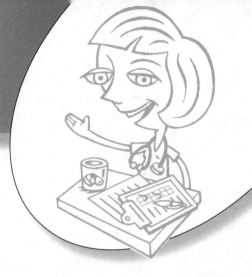

Introduction

After making an appointment, providing information about our medical insurer, and paying a token amount called a copay, rarely do we give a second thought on how practitioners, hospitals, and others in the healthcare industry get paid. Our copay is a fraction of the total cost of our visit. Medical insurers pay the bulk of our medical costs—but not before our healthcare provider submits an insurance claim along with supporting documents to justify the treatment we received during the visit.

Only if the claim is approved will the healthcare provider get paid. This appears to be a well-oiled efficient system for covering medical expenses. At least that's true from the patient's perspective. It can be a nightmare for a healthcare provider who cares for hundreds of patients daily with each having a different medical coverage and requiring a different treatment. Imagine trying to assemble a detailed bill with different supporting documents for each of the hundreds of patients treated by a healthcare provider every day—and tomorrow there are another hundred patients arriving. Your healthcare provider can easily be in a financial bind if there isn't a constant, dependable stream of reimbursements from insurers. Your healthcare provider pays the cost of the medical and administrative staff, rent, utilities, and vendors who provided medical supplies and pharmaceuticals used to treat you. These expenses are paid before your healthcare provider is reimbursed by the medical insurer for your visit. Reimbursements stop flowing when insurers deny claims or delay processing them, and many times this is caused by medical billing and coding errors. Honest— and sometimes dumb—mistakes cause insurers to withhold reimbursements until the healthcare provider submits a correct claim.

Healthcare providers are on a financial tightrope balanced only by the stream of insurance reimbursements. They are trained to care for patients—not to navigate the maze of insurance rules and regulations.

Healthcare providers rely on medical insurance specialists who know how to prepare claims and supporting documents to ensure that medical insurers approve claims—and keep reimbursements flowing.

The medical insurance specialists must:

- Thoroughly understand healthcare economics
- Understand the ethical and legal aspects of healthcare and insurance
- Be well versed in medical terminology and procedures
- Know medical office procedures
- Master procedure coding
- Grasp the details of medical insurance plans
- Take command of the insurance claim cycle
- Skillfully handle claims disputes
- Be a whiz at using medical management computer software
- And much more

This can be overwhelming but doable because there are proven techniques that medical insurance specialists use every day to tackle what seem like insurmountable problems. *Medical Billing and Coding Demystified* shows you those techniques and how to apply them in real-life clinical situations.

You might be a little apprehensive to pursue a medical insurance specialist's position. Medical billing and coding can be mystifying; however, it will become demystified as you read this book. By the end of this book you'll be able to step up to a medical insurance specialist's responsibilities and begin to solve practically any problem that comes your way.

A Look Inside

Medical billing and coding is challenging unless you follow the proven approach that is used in *Medical Billing and Coding Demystified*. In this second edition, focus is on ICD-10CM. Topics are presented in an order in which many medical insurance specialists like to learn them—starting with the basics and then gradually moving on to techniques used every day to ensure insurance reimbursements steadily flow into some of our nation's leading medical facilities.

Each chapter follows a time-tested formula that first explains techniques in an easy-to-read style and then shows how you can use it in the real-world healthcare environment. You can then test your knowledge at the end of each chapter to be sure that you have mastered medical insurance specialist skills. There is little room for you to go adrift.

Chapter 1 Introduction to Medical Billing and Coding

Did you ever wonder how physicians and hospitals get paid? Probably not because in the United States, we normally don't pay for medical care directly; instead our medical insurer pays for it. We simply visit our physician's office or the hospital and provide information about our health insurance. We might be asked to pay a token amount called a copay, but that's a fraction of the total medical bill. In this chapter, you'll be introduced to the business aspects of healthcare.

Chapter 2 Ethical and Legal Aspects of Medical Billing

Medical insurance specialists work with patients' confidential medical records and therefore must adhere to ethical and legal standards common to the medical profession. This chapter discusses those standards and how to comply with them.

Chapter 3 Medical Terminology and Procedures

As a medical insurance specialist, you'll need to become fluent in medical terminology in order to properly code medical procedures to prepare medical bills for a healthcare facility. Learning medical terminology might seem overwhelming at first. However, in this chapter you'll learn the secret that will make understanding medical technology come natural to you.

Chapter 4 Medical Office Procedures

While sitting in a waiting room you watch doctors and the healthcare team go about their business—all the time scratching your head wondering what they are doing. As a medical insurance specialist, you'll be part of that healthcare team. In this chapter, you'll learn the responsibilities of each team member, how they interact with each other, and procedures commonly used in every medical practice.

Chapter 5 Introduction to Procedural Coding

It's time to learn how billing codes are used to pay for medical procedures. There are countless medical procedures and services that healthcare professionals provide to patients every day, and each is charged separately. It is an administrative nightmare—that is, if it wasn't for a coding system that streamlines claims processing so that computers can handle most claims with little human intervention. This chapter introduces you to medical billing codes and ICD-10-CM and walks you through the steps necessary to code a medical claim.

Chapter 6 Introduction to Insurance Plans

Healthcare providers will look to you as a medical insurance specialist to guide them through the maze of health insurance plans to ensure that a steady stream of reimbursements flow into the practice. This chapter shows you how to find your way through the maze of health insurance plans and gives you the foundation to advise healthcare providers on how to ensure that reimbursements are not denied.

Chapter 7 The Insurance Claim Cycle

Processing medical claims is a mission-critical function for every physician practice, hospital, outpatient clinic, hospice, and laboratory. Any delay in processing directly impacts the bottom line because it delays payment. In this chapter, you'll learn about the insurance claim cycle and about how to avoid unnecessary delays in receiving reimbursement from medical insurers. You'll also learn about different types of healthcare coverage that the medical insurance specialists must deal with daily.

Chapter 8 Billing and Coding Errors: How to Avoid Them

A constant, dependable stream of reimbursements from insurers is the blood that keeps a medical practice and a healthcare facility alive. Reimbursements stop flowing when insurers deny claims or delay processing them. And coding and billing errors are the major reasons why this happens. The medical insurance specialist's responsibility is to keep reimbursements flowing by making sure all claims are error free before they are sent to an insurer for processing. In this chapter, you'll learn the most common mistakes that cause insurers to reject claims.

Chapter 9 Strategies for Handling Claim Disputes

Every insurance claim undergoes an adjudication process during which a claims examiner determines if the claim is covered by the terms of the patient's insurance policy. If the claim is denied, the healthcare provider—and the patient—can appeal the claims examiner's decision. In this chapter, you'll learn how to resolve claim disputes without going through an appeal. You'll also learn how to develop a winning strategy for an appeal.

Chapter 10 Medical Transportation

Patients who are unable to come themselves to the healthcare facility are transported by other means. Transportation is divided into two groups: emergency transportation and nonemergency transportation. Emergency transportation typically includes emergency medical service (EMS) providers in the form of a ground or air ambulance. Nonemergency transportation includes wheelchair vans, taxi cabs, automobile, and buses. Health insurers typically reimburse for medical transportation services if required by the patient's medical condition. Medical transportation services are billed separately from other medical services such as those generated by hospitals and practitioners. You'll learn about how to bill for medical transportation in this chapter.

Chapter 11 Medical Practice

There are a lot of activities that take place while the patient is waiting to see the practitioner. The patient is unaware of many of these tasks. The patient arrives and registers at the receptionist's desk. Typically, the receptionist asks for the patient's name and then enters the patient's name into the computer to bring up information about the patient, which usually includes information about the patient's most recent health insurer. In this chapter, you'll learn about medical practice including reimbursement guidelines that assist the practitioner care for the patient.

Chapter 12 Medical Billing Software Programs and Systems

Nearly 75% of medical insurance claims and all Medicare claims are processed electronically using a computer program resulting in 98% of those claims being reimbursed within 30 days. Today medical insurance specialists must be as well versed in medical management computer programs as they are in medical insurance. In this chapter, you'll learn about computer technology and how to perform common tasks using one of the most widely adopted medical management computer programs in the industry.

Chapter 13 Finding Employment in the Healthcare Industry

Finding your first job as a medical insurance specialist is a challenge because you'll need to convince a prospective employer to bring you on board his or her healthcare team. Medical insurance specialists are in demand by healthcare providers in private practice, healthcare facilities, insurance companies, and private industry that need someone to help them manage their medical benefits program. In this chapter, you'll learn strategies for job searching and techniques for preparing and submitting resumes and interviewing with prospective employers.

Medical Billing and Coding
DeMYSTiFieD

chapter 1

Introduction to Medical Billing and Coding

LEARNING OBJECTIVES

1. The Business of Healthcare
2. The Economics of Healthcare
3. The Money Game
4. The Marketing Game
5. A Brief Look Back at Healthcare
6. Medical Insurance Specialist

KEY TERMS

Blue Cross and Blue Shield

Compulsory National Health
  Insurance

For-Profit and Not-For-Profit
Healthcare Charges

In Comes the Insurance Industry

Medical Insurance as a Wage

Medical Insurance Specialist

Medical Insurance Specialists
  Certification

Medicare and Medicaid

ObamaCare: The Affordable Care Act

Paying Bills

Qualifications for Medical Insurance
  Specialists

Reducing the Number of Healthcare
  Providers

Squeezing Out Waste

Supply and Demand

The Money Trail

The Pricing Games

The Uninsured

1. The Business of Healthcare

Did you ever wonder how physicians and hospitals get paid? Probably not, because in the United States we normally don't pay for medical care directly; instead our medical insurer pays for it. We simply visit our physician's office or the hospital and provide information about our health insurance. We might be asked to pay a token amount called *co-pay*, but that's a fraction of the total medical bill.

After treatment, healthcare providers, including physicians, hospitals, and other healthcare facilities, submit our medical bill to the medical insurer. If the bill is approved, the medical insurer pays our healthcare provider directly for all or a portion of our services.

This appears to be a well-oiled, efficient system for covering medical expenses, at least from the patient's perspective. However, this system can be a nightmare for healthcare providers who care for hundreds of patients daily with each patient having a different medical coverage and requiring a different treatment.

Medical insurers reimburse healthcare providers according to necessary procedures performed on the patient. It is up to the healthcare provider to supply the medical insurer with supporting evidence that the procedure was necessary. The healthcare provider doesn't get paid unless the supporting documents accompany the bill. This sounds logical until you realize that each health insurer requires different types of supporting documents.

Imagine trying to assemble a detailed bill with different supporting documents for each of the hundreds of patients treated by a healthcare provider every day. It can become a nightmare, and any error will delay payment.

Fortunately, healthcare providers can rely on medical billing and coding professionals known as *medical insurance specialists,* who know how to prepare bills and supporting documents so that medical insurers can authorize payment.

Throughout this book you'll learn the skills necessary to become a medical insurance specialist. We'll begin in this chapter with a brief introduction to the concepts of medical billing and coding.

2. The Economics of Healthcare

Our method of paying for healthcare has evolved over the past century (see the section A Brief Look Back at Healthcare later in this chapter) and continues to evolve today where slick marketing techniques normally reserved for selling soap and automobiles are used to sell prescription medication, medical tests, and hospital services to prospective patients.

You've probably seen radio and television commercials touting the benefits of one hospital over another or how a $3,000 body scan can identify the infancy of a disease so that you can be treated before the disease spread further. Pharmaceutical firms advertise their latest drugs directly to patients although the drug can only be purchased with a prescription from a healthcare provider.

Economics is the driving force that pushes the healthcare industry to aggressively go after the patient as the consumer of its products and services. It is a branch of social science that deals with the production, distribution, and consumption of goods and services.

Many of us don't consider health a consumer product or service like buying groceries or an automobile. Yet, healthcare is a business with a sole purpose to provide products and services in exchange for money.

For-Profit and Not-For-Profit

Healthcare providers are divided into two economic categories: for-profit and not-for-profit.

- A **for-profit healthcare provider** charges fees that cover expenses and return a profit. Profit is money collected by the healthcare provider that exceeds expenses and is distributed to its owners as a reward for investing money in the business. An owner can be a physician, a group of physicians, or anyone who invests money to start the healthcare business.

- A **not-for-profit healthcare provider** charges fees that cover expenses only. Theoretically, not for profit healthcare providers do not receive extra income. There isn't a profit and there aren't any investors. Not-for-profit healthcare providers strive to bring in enough money to cover expenses and to have enough money in hand to handle unexpected expenses—a kind of emergency fund.

Supply and Demand

The healthcare industry is governed by the economic rule of **supply and demand**. This rule states simply that a demand by consumers for products and services will cause someone to provide those products and services. If there is no demand, then no one will invest time and money making the product or providing the service.

For example, a town of 100 people has a demand for services of a physician. However, the demand is too small to attract a physician because there aren't enough unwell people to make it profitable for a physician to set up a practice in the town.

As the town grows to 5,000 people, the demand for healthcare services increases to a level that makes it profitable for one physician to open a practice in town. Still there aren't sufficient unwell people to support a hospital. A town of 50,000 or more might be needed to attract a hospital.

A for-profit healthcare provider enters a market when demand is enough to return a profit and withdraws from the market when demand becomes unprofitable. However, not-for-profit healthcare providers usually remain in unprofitable markets because they receive funding from government agencies or charities.

The Money Trail

You've probably heard the story about the hospital that charged a patient $1 for an aspirin when the local pharmacy sells a bottle of aspirin for 69 cents. This is true. The hospital probably paid a penny for the aspirin but charged a dollar to bring in additional revenue.

Revenue is money that is paid to a healthcare provider. Healthcare providers seek to have as many revenue streams as possible. A *revenue stream* is a product or service that is sold to bring in money. For example, the parking lot fee at the hospital is a revenue stream and so is the rental fee for telephones and televisions. And of course providing the patient with aspirin and other medications is another revenue stream.

The amount of revenue that can be generated by a revenue stream depends on the amount of money the healthcare provider charges for a product or service—charging $2 for an aspirin brings in more money (greater revenue stream) than charging $1 for the aspirin.

Healthcare providers try to maximize the money generated by each revenue stream in order to provide the cash needed to run their operation. This is true regardless of whether the healthcare provider is for-profit or not-for-profit.

Healthcare Charges

A *fee* is the price a healthcare provider charges for a product or service. This is similar to the sticker price on a car. Each healthcare provider sets the fee based on supply and demand although some healthcare providers adjust the fee based on the patient's ability to pay.

When a lot of healthcare providers supply the same product or service, fees are competitive in order to attract new patients and to retain current patients. *Competitive* means that fees for the same product or service are relatively around the same amount. This is like all Ford dealers in the area selling the same model car at about the same price.

Fees are less competitive when there is a high demand for a product or service and there are few healthcare providers supplying it. Typically, the high demand encourages other healthcare providers to supply the product or service resulting in a competitive price.

Remember that fees are equivalent to prices. We see pricing being adjusted according to supply and demand in grocery stores or at the gas pump, but rarely do we see this happening in healthcare because our medical insurer pays our medical bills.

The fee a medical insurer pays is not necessarily the fee seen on our medical bill. This is like the sticker price on a car. You probably pay less than the sticker price. Medical insurers typically pay the allowed charge or the usual, customary, and reasonable fee for a product or service within the specific section of the country.

Let's say that your hospital charges a dollar for an aspirin even though other hospitals in the area normally charge 40 cents. Your medical insurer pays the hospital 40 cents—not the dollar. The hospital has the option to accept the 40 cents as full payment or send you a bill for remaining 60 cents.

Healthcare providers sometimes find themselves in a dilemma. In some cases, the amount that the medical insurer pays doesn't provide a sufficient financial incentive for the healthcare provider to supply the product or provide the service.

The healthcare provider can send the patient a bill for the difference between the original bill and the amount the medical insurer reimbursed; however, the patient may complain and find another healthcare provider.

Furthermore, the patient may be unable to pay the difference. This leaves the healthcare provider to seek legal recourse against the patient, which is expensive and may become public resulting in a loss of other patients who could feel that the healthcare provider is overcharging them.

In these situations, the healthcare provider might appeal the partial reimbursement to the medical insurer. An *appeal* is a request for the medical insurer to take a second look at the claim. Alternatively, the healthcare provider might simply accept the partial reimbursement as payment in full.

Paying Bills

Healthcare providers need to receive reimbursement for medical insurance claims in a timely manner; otherwise they won't be able to pay their bills. This is like you receiving your paycheck each pay period. If you miss a pay period, you may not be able to pay your bills.

Remember the last visit you made to your healthcare provider? You were greeted by a receptionist and then shown into the examination room by a healthcare professional such as a nurse or a medical assistant. The office was well stocked with various medical equipment and supplies. The healthcare provider might have given you an injection of medication following the examination. Once completed, the office staff prepared and submitted your medical claim to the insurance company.

Your healthcare provider is responsible for paying the medical and administrative staff, rent, utilities, and vendors who provided medical supplies and pharmaceuticals used to treat you. These expenses are paid before your medical insurer reimburses the healthcare provider for your visit. The healthcare provider must supply funds to cover expenses until payment is received from your medical insurer.

These funds come from various sources

- Payments from previous medical insurance claims.
- Short-term bank loans.
- Profit from payment received from previous visits.
- Investors who provide funds for a chance to share in the profits.
- Personal funds of the healthcare providers.

3. The Money Game

Medical insurers make money by investing premiums. A *premium* is what you pay for medical coverage. The medical insurer gambles it will earn more money from investments than it will pay in medical insurance claims.

Let's say that you pay a $100-per-month premium for medical insurance or $1,200 per year. You're in pretty good health and didn't have to visit your physician during the year. This means that your medical insurer has $1,200 since it didn't need to reimburse a healthcare provider for medical expenses.

Over the course of the year, the insurer invested the $1,200 and earned 10%—that's $12 per month or $120 for the year. Investments can range from overnight loans to a bank to investing in a shopping mall.

The medical insurer gambles that you and its other policyholders as a group won't incur an average of $1,200 each worth of medical expenses in a year. The gamble pays off if the medical insurer properly sets the premium based on the probability that a particular group of people will require a specific level of healthcare during the year. This simply means that, for example, as a group, racecar drivers will pay more for healthcare coverage than office workers because racecar drivers have a higher probability of requiring medical care than office workers.

Don't be concerned about premiums and probability because you won't use it. However, you should be familiar with the concept of time value of money, which is the principle used by medical insurers when investing premiums. *Time value of money* means that the medical insurer (or anyone who invests) makes more money from its investments the longer the money is invested. In our example, the medical insurer makes $12 per month for each month as it invests your $1,200 premium.

Suppose a healthcare provider submits a $1,200 claim to a medical insurer for a patient's visit. The medical insurer takes a month to process the claim (and earns $12 from the investment). The medical insurer asks the healthcare provider to submit additional supporting documents, which takes another month (and earns $12 from the investment). Once the claim is approved, another month passes until the healthcare provider receives cash (and the medical insurer earns another $12 from the investment).

Notice that the medical insurer in this example earned $36 by not paying the claim within 30 days of receiving the paperwork from the healthcare provider. In practice, the longer the medical insurer delays payment, the more money the medical insurer earns from its investments.

However, the longer payment is delayed, the more the patient's visit costs the healthcare provider. In a negative cash flow, the healthcare provider is paying interest and bank fees on loans. In a **positive cash flow**, the healthcare provider is forgoing earning money on investments to pay expenses.

Conflicts arise between medical insurers and healthcare providers over the timeliness of payment. Some healthcare providers feel some medical insurers are needlessly delaying payment in order to earn more money from investments. Some medical insurers feel some healthcare providers are performing needless procedures to increase their claims and therefore claims must be carefully documented and reviewed, which is time-consuming.

The Pricing Games

A healthcare provider can charge any fee for a procedure. However, that doesn't mean the healthcare provider will be paid that fee. In theory the fee for a product or service reflects what the consumer of the product or service is willing to pay. For example, a car dealer may charge $100,000 for an automobile, but few—if any—consumers will be willing to pay that amount for the car.

Healthcare providers set their fees based on how medical insurers reimburse the healthcare provider. The medical insurer is a sophisticated buyer—someone who does homework to determine a fair market price for a product or service. This is like you researching for car prices before negotiating a price with a car dealer.

Medical insurers study the market carefully and calculate the cost for performing every medical procedure and survey healthcare providers throughout the country to determine the normal fee for each procedure. This information is used by medical insurers to set the reimbursement to healthcare providers.

Squeezing Out Waste

Medical costs are skyrocketing. There are numerous reasons given by the medical industry for this rise in fees. Some reasons are true and others are half-truths. Regardless, medical insurers devise ways to reduce reimbursements paid to healthcare providers.

A widely used method is to negotiate with healthcare providers a fixed reimbursement for commonly performed procedures. Healthcare providers who reach terms with a medical insurer become a member of the medical insurer's network of healthcare providers.

Since reimbursement is fixed, medical insurers lower their risk of high reimbursement and therefore can offer better terms if patients receive a procedure from a healthcare provider who is within the medical insurer's network rather than from a healthcare provider who is out-of-network.

The terms of the agreement with healthcare providers reflect fees that the healthcare provider will be reimbursed by the medical insurer. For example, between 80% and 100% of the negotiated fee is reimbursed if the healthcare provider is in-network as compared with 60% of the providers fees if the healthcare provider is out-of-network. The patient pays the difference.

The patient has a financial incentive for using only in-network healthcare providers. Healthcare providers expect to see an appreciable increase in their business if they join the network. However, the healthcare provider might have to lower fees. The medical insurer can reduce the increase in medical cost by negotiating fixed fees, which enables the insurer to offer better terms to employers. In turn this attracts more business, generating additional premiums that can be invested.

Some medical insurers run health maintenance organizations (HMOs). In many cases, these are healthcare facilities run and operated by the insurer and provide it the opportunity to reduce the expenses of operating the facility (called *operating expenses*) by negotiating better prices with suppliers. Patients who use HMOs don't pay anything for medical procedures other than their premium.

4. The Marketing Game

The business of healthcare has undergone a dramatic change in recent years. Healthcare providers can no longer set fees freely because medical insurers may not pay those fees. A healthcare provider can refuse to accept terms set forth by medical insurers; however, there is a high probability that their patients will find a healthcare provider who accepts the medical insurer's terms rather than pay more than is required for a medical procedure.

Many healthcare providers are feeling the squeeze and seeing their incomes drop compared with the time before medical insurers negotiated special terms with healthcare providers. As a result, some healthcare providers have turned to marketing techniques traditionally used by consumer-product companies to increase their business—and their income.

No doubt you've heard commercials for hospitals that tout how well they rank among other local hospitals. They go straight to the patient for new business rather than rely on physicians. Traditionally hospitals pitched their services only to physicians who then sent their patients to the hospital for medical procedures. The patients had little choice because their physician was usually associated with one or maybe two local hospitals.

Practically all hospitals have negotiated terms with most medical insurers, making them an in-network healthcare provider. This means that patients receive the best possible fee according to their medical coverage regardless of the hospital. Likewise, many physicians who are in-network are associated with in-network hospitals. The patient now has the capability to choose which hospital will perform the medical procedure.

Hospitals use the airwaves and print media to convince patients that their medical facility is better than other local hospitals. Furthermore, hospitals and other medical facilities create new or enhanced services and then try to persuade patients to buy those services.

For example, in some areas of the country, medical facilities tell patients to undergo a full body scan to find tumors and other abnormalities long before symptoms appear. The full body scan is priced at the cost of a 3-week family vacation. The scan is probably not covered by medical insurance because it isn't medically justified. That is, a physician didn't recognize symptoms first before ordering the diagnostic test.

Consumer marketing techniques overcome this problem by convincing patients to directly pay the cost of the procedure—your life might depend on it. They even offer financing plans. Physicians point out that in rare cases this might be true, but for most people the full body scan is an unnecessary medical procedure unless the patient shows symptoms of a disease.

In fact, physicians have said that the body scan is likely to find abnormalities such as growths that normally occur in most people but have no negative effect. However, the patient is likely to incur additional medical procedures if these abnormalities are revealed by the full body scan. And this means more business—and more income—for the facility that performed the full body scan and for physicians who are associated with that facility. Medical insurers likely cover those additional procedures because the discovery of the abnormalities provided the medical reason for further procedures.

Healthcare providers are starting to use consumer marketing to increase the number of procedures they perform since a price increase no longer guarantees them a higher income.

5. A Brief Look Back at Healthcare

Now that you have an idea of how the healthcare industry works today, we'll take a look back in time and see how the healthcare system in the United States has evolved. Before 1920, the cost of medical treatment was low, simply because medical technology and procedures were primitive compared with today's standards. Most treatments—including surgery—were performed at home using only the basics of medications.

These were the early years of modern medicine during which physicians were learning about bacteriology, antisepsis, and immunology. Scientists were improving medical technology by introducing the blood pressure machine and X-rays.

Most people had very low medical expenses. Interestingly, the most costly effect of getting ill was loss of wages. Ill people simply didn't get paid. Families purchased health insurance; however, coverage was much different than today's medical coverage. Health insurance in those days was called *sick insurance*. Sick insurance didn't cover medical expenses. Instead, sick insurance covered lost wages much like today's disability insurance.

Insurance companies didn't offer what we know of as health insurance because of the high risk of fraud. An unhealthy person might purchase a medical insurance policy claiming he was healthy. The premium would be set based on a healthy person. The insurer would then lose money when the person submitted the claims for procedures undergone by an unhealthy person. This sounds absurd by today's standards because there are now medical procedures in place to determine the health of a person, but before 1920 being "sick" was vague. There wasn't a single definition of sick that the medical industry and the insurance industry could agree on.

Compulsory National Health Insurance

Although medical costs were negligible, people before 1920 became sick at even a greater rate than today because of the primitive nature of medical knowledge. Government leaders in the United States and in Europe realized there was a need for true health insurance—not sick insurance—because of new and improved medical techniques and the growth of drugs to treat disease.

Many European countries adopted compulsory national health insurance that covered the medical expenses of everyone in the country. With pressure from the **American Association for Labor Legislation** (AALL), efforts were put forth for legislation to create a compulsory health insurance. It failed for two reasons.

First, lawmakers didn't see an immediate need because medical expenses were very low. However, the major reason for failure was because physicians and the insurance industry campaigned against the law. Physicians felt that the government would limit their fees. The insurance industry saw health insurance as an unmanageable risk. Furthermore, the law would have prohibited the insurance companies from offering burial insurance, which was a large part of their business.

The expectations of government leaders were realized. Medical expenses rose between 1920 and 1930 as medical procedures improved and newly discovered drugs gave the ill/ailing people realistic hope of being cured. The ill people were treated in hospitals instead of homes because hospitals were kept clean and antiseptic, which increased the use of hospitals—and increased medical expenses.

There was a shift in the population from farms to cities. People who lived on a farm typically were more self-sufficient than those living in the cities because help was miles away. The influx to the cities resulted in families living closer together in smaller living quarters. This bred disease. If one person became ill, the entire family would be ill and need medical treatment. In turn, medical expenses increased. The public's attitude toward medicine changed also. Medicine was seen as a precise, effective science that could cure many ailments. There was a great improvement in medical care by 1930.

Reducing the Number of Healthcare Providers

Supply and demand also increased the price of medical care. The **American Medical Association** (AMA) established requirements for practicing medicine that included graduation from an accredited medical school. Medical schools had to toughen admission requirements, raise fees, and institute strict graduation requirements. The result was a drop in the number of physicians practicing medicine and a rise in medical fees.

The **American College of Surgeons** organized to set standards for surgeons and hospitals. Hospitals had to meet those standards before being accredited. Some hospitals didn't meet these standards and therefore were not accredited.

In the late 1920s, an investigation was launched to look at the rise in medical expenses. A committee was formed called the **Committee on the Cost of Medical Care**. It discovered that 5% of an urban family's income was spent for nonhospital medical care. This rose to 13% if a family member was hospitalized.

Blue Cross and Blue Shield

The high cost of hospitalization and relatively low family wages resulted in many unpaid hospital bills. In an effort to rope in hospital bills, a group of

Dallas teachers negotiated an arrangement with Baylor University Hospital for prepaid hospital service—21 days of hospitalization for $6. The deal capped the cost of their hospital stay and guaranteed Baylor University Hospital payment and a steady income.

The concept of prepaid hospitalization spread. Many hospitals joined together to offer their own hospitalization coverage. This effort also reduced competition among hospitals. The American Hospital Association brought together all these plans into one plan called *Blue Cross*.

Grouping together these plans in one plan reduced price competition among the plans and gave subscribers the choice of using a breadth of physicians and hospitals rather than just those who participated in the smaller plans. States granted Blue Cross tax-exempt status and freed it from regulations that governed the insurance industry. They did this because Blue Cross was seen as an organization that benefited society as a whole.

Blue Cross paid subscriber's hospital bills, but not physician bills. Physicians were not in a rush to join a similar prepayment service because the prepayment service would interfere with income and interfere with their relationship with patients. Furthermore, an individual physician would no longer be able to set prices.

By the 1930s, physicians saw the writing on the wall. Prepaid hospitalization plans became popular among their patients—and their patients wanted a prepaid plan for physician care. Blue Cross considered expanding coverage to include physicians. Lawmakers rekindled interest in compulsory health insurance.

Physicians decided to offer their own prepaid policy to cover physician services. The AMA developed guidelines for these plans that fought off compulsory health insurance. The guidelines specified that voluntary plans must be under the supervision of a physician and gave physicians the right to set prices for services based on the patient's ability to pay. The first physician service prepayment plan opened in 1939 and was called the *California Physicians' Service* (CPS). Subscribers paid $1.70 per month if they earned less than $3,000 per year. Prepayment plans caught on throughout the country. In 1946, these plans were organized into one group called *Blue Shield*.

With Blue Shield, patients had to pay physicians the difference between the price the physician charged for the service and the money reimbursed to the physician by Blue Shield. This meant that physicians were free to charge whatever they wanted—many charged less to low-income subscribers than to their more wealthy patients.

In Comes the Insurance Industry

The health insurance industry matured between 1940 and 1960. The success of Blue Cross and Blue Shield proved to the insurance industry that there was a way to offer medical insurance without being exposed to widespread fraud as the insurance industry originally believed. Improvements in medicine during this period also increased the demand for medical care.

The medical industry focused on offering medical insurance to employed workers who were traditionally young and healthy but without health insurance. The health insurance market grew 700% between 1940 and 1950.

Blue Cross and Blue Shield set policy rates using the community rating system because they were not-for-profit organizations. The **community rating system** required that the same premium be charged regardless of whether the subscriber was healthy or ill.

Alternative health insurance companies used the experience rating system to set premiums. In the **experience rating system**, the premium was set based on the claims the subscriber submitted. That is, a healthy subscriber paid a lower premium than an unhealthy subscriber. Insurance companies used the experienced rating system to their advantage by targeting groups of healthy people who subscribed to Blue Cross and Blue Shield. The experienced rating system enabled insurance companies to offer a lower premium to these groups than the groups paid to Blue Cross and Blue Shield for the same coverage. It didn't take long for the insurance companies to have more subscribers than Blue Cross and Blue Shield.

Medical Insurance as a Wage

During World War II, Congress passed the **1942 Stabilization Act** that instituted wage and price controls. Employers were permitted to give employees a limited raise in wages. One of the objectives of this act was to reduce competition among employers for employees. There was a shortage of workers because many of them were in the armed services fighting the war.

Therefore, an employer couldn't offer more money for a worker to change jobs. However, employers were permitted to offer insurance plans. This began the practice of employers offering health insurance as a benefit to employees. Insurance companies saw this as an opportunity to sell medical insurance, to be offered by employers, as a benefit to their employees.

Forerunners of today's healthcare insurance got a boost from the labor movement and two legal rulings. In the 1940s, the United States was a manufacturing economy where many workers worked in factories and belonged to a labor union. Labor unions negotiated employment contracts with employers for union members.

The **War Labor Board**, which was a federal agency that oversaw labor during World War II, ruled that employers could not cancel or modify group health insurance during the term of the contract. This meant that workers whose employers provided medical insurance would guarantee coverage until the union contract expired.

In 1949, the **National Labor Relations Board**, which oversaw labor after the War Labor Board was disbanded following the end of the war, ruled that medical insurance was part of an employee's wages and therefore granted the right to negotiate medical insurance benefits to the union. This rule recognized that medical insurance is part of the wage package offered to employees by an employer and created the de facto employer-based health insurance system that we still have today.

The federal government encouraged employers to offer medical insurance benefits to employees by making medical insurance premiums exempt from payroll tax. Traditionally, employers paid a payroll tax on wages paid to employees. Since medical insurance was considered part of an employee's wage, it therefore would have been taxed if not exempted.

Likewise, employees had to pay tax on their wages. Therefore, the medical insurance premium paid by the employer on behalf of an employee was considered a wage on which the employee must pay a payroll tax. However in 1943, the federal government ruled that this was not taxable income. This was ratified in a revision to the **Internal Revenue Code** in 1954.

The Uninsured

Three-quarters of all people in the United States were covered by health insurance in 1958. The United States managed to develop a privately funded and operated health insurance system that was favorable to subscribers, employers, and healthcare providers.

However, there was a problem with private health insurance. Only workers and their families were covered. The unemployed could purchase a health insurance policy, but most couldn't afford the premium. Many of these people were unwell or elderly, which increased their risk of becoming ill. Medical insurance companies priced premiums based on an analysis of past medical reimbursements. Those who were at a higher risk of becoming ill would incur higher medical expenses; therefore, they were charged higher premiums than workers.

The solution was national health insurance. Government leaders realized that there was a large opposition to national health insurance. Rather than fight a battle that had been lost many times, government leaders proposed government-sponsored health insurance that provided medical coverage to the elderly—people older than 65 years. Most opponents agreed with the plan. That is, all but one opponent. The AMA feared that government-sponsored health insurance would encourage patients to request unnecessary medical services and therefore overload the medical system. Government leaders recognized this potential and limited government-sponsored health insurance to only hospitals.

Medicare and Medicaid

By the mid-1960s, the political climate changed in the United States—and so did opposition to national health insurance. In 1965, Congress passed the **Social Security Act**, which created Medicare and Medicaid.

Medicare is government-sponsored health insurance paid for by a payroll tax that was divided into two parts. The first part was called *Part A* and provided hospital insurance for the elderly. People older than 65 years were automatically enrolled in Part A of Medicare. The second part was called *Part B* and provided medical insurance for services provided by physicians. Part B was a supplemental medical insurance that reimbursed physicians based on the physician's usual, customary, and reasonable rates. Furthermore, physicians sent their full bill to the patient. The patient then forwarded it to Medicare for reimbursement. This meant that physicians could set their fees according to how much a patient could afford to pay. The patient had to pay the entire physician's bill even if Medicare reimbursed the patient less than the full bill.

Medicare provided medical insurance for the elderly; however, there were still people who were not employed and not elderly but were not covered by medical insurance. The federal government created Medicaid to address this population.

Medicaid is a joint program operated by the federal and state governments to provide medical insurance for the indigent. The federal government gives states a Medicaid payment based on the state's per capita income compared with the national per capita income.

The federal government provides a definition of **indigent** by specifying minimum eligibility and benefit standards, the Federal Poverty Guidelines. Each state can broaden these standards. This means that Medicaid covers every person who meets the federal government's defined standard. Those who don't qualify may still qualify for Medicaid if they meet their state's Medicaid standard. However, state Medicaid standards differ from state to state.

The number of Medicare subscribers grew to a level that stretched the government's capability of funding the program. In 1983, the government changed the way healthcare providers were reimbursed. Instead of reimbursing at the usual and customary rates, the government reimbursed based on a fixed fee schedule.

ObamaCare: The Affordable Care Act

In 2010, the Affordable Care Act was passed by Congress and signed into law to significantly overhaul the healthcare system in the United States. The Affordable Care Act along with the Health Care and Education Reconciliation Act became the most significant healthcare change since the creation of Medicare and Medicaid.

The Affordable Care Act's goal is to reduce the overall cost of healthcare in the United States primarily by making health insurance available to everyone—and requiring everyone to be covered by health insurance.

Insurance is a gamble for both the insurer and the person who purchases it. All of us are at risk for an event that can negatively impact our lives. For example, a car can be destroyed in an accident, fire or flood can make our home unlivable, and we can fall sick, exposing us to high medical expenses.

Purchasing insurance is a way to mitigate the risk—not lowering or preventing the risk from occurring. That is, your car can still be involved in an accident, your house can be destroyed by fire or flood, and you will get ill at some point. However, expenses associated with these negative events will be paid for in part or whole by the insurer if you pay a regular amount of money called a *premium*.

In essence, you are betting a small amount of money (premium) that you will experience the negative event and the insurer is betting that you won't—or that most of insured people will not experience the negative event. Premiums collected by the insurer are used to pay the claims of the insured who incurred expenses relative to the negative event; however, those are likely very few compared with the insured who paid premiums and did not experience a negative event. Excess premiums are invested by the insurer to bring in increased revenue and profit.

Not all people in the United States are covered by health insurance. Employees are offered health insurance through their employer; however, the relatively high cost of offering health insurance causes smaller business to offer high cost, limited coverage insurance to employees—or no health insurance coverage.

Those not covered by an employer's health insurance have the option of purchasing individual health insurance policies; however, these policies are expensive and may have a high deductible, leaving the insured to pay for all but catastrophic illnesses. As a result, they forgo purchasing health insurance.

Typically, those not covered by health insurance do not qualify for Medicare or Medicaid. That is, they fall through the health insurance gap. The uninsured forgo medical care when they are ill, which can lead to more serious illnesses and increased care costs. Medical care for the uninsured is typically provided by the emergency department, which is one of the most costly forms of medical care. The cost of care is usually paid by the local government through the form of charity care. The patient pays nothing.

The Affordable Care Act is designed to fill most if not all of this gap by:

- Requiring everyone to purchase health insurance otherwise the government will impose a fine.
- Creating online health insurance exchanges that provide a one-stop marketplace for health insurers to offer individual health insurance policies providing a tool for individuals and businesses to compare policies and prices.
- Establishing minimum coverage for all health insurance policies such as preventive care.
- Restricting insurance company practices that open gaps in medical coverage such as no coverage of preexisting conditions.
- Providing a government subsidy for premiums based on a person or business income. The government will pay some or all of the premium for those who are unable to afford purchasing a health insurance policy.
- Lowering requirements for participating in Medicaid, which enabled more people to participate in the program.
- Streamlining Medicare payments by adopting a bundled payment practice rather than fee-for-service. Healthcare providers are paid for a defined episode, such as a knee replacement, rather than paid for each service related to the knee replacement.

6. Medical Insurance Specialist

The financial stability of healthcare providers is tied to a steady, dependable flow of payments from medical insurance companies and the government for services provided to subscribers. There are thousands of medical insurers, each having their own procedures for receiving, approving, and paying claims. Healthcare providers hire medical insurance specialists to submit claims, respond to inquiries from medical insurers, and follow up on overdue payments.

Throughout this book you'll learn the skills and techniques to become a medical insurance specialist. Medical insurance specialists are employed by hospitals, medical offices, and other healthcare providers who treat patients.

Medical insurance specialists must know claims processing and billing regulations and know how to code bills based on the procedure the healthcare provider performed on the patient. The medical insurance specialist must also know how to appeal claims that are rejected by a medical insurance company or claims medical insurers partially pay.

In this chapter you learned how medical insurers try to rope in medical expenses and in doing so create extra work for healthcare providers, such as requiring preauthorization by the medical insurer before the healthcare provider performs certain procedures on the patient. And posttreatment reports must be submitted to the medical insurer following the procedure. The medical insurance specialist is typically the person responsible for getting the preauthorization and preparing and submitting posttreatment reports.

Medical insurance specialists specialize in one or more of the following areas:

- **Claims benefit advisor**. Provides expert advice to healthcare providers, malpractice lawyers, and liability insurance companies
- **Coding specialist**. Prepares claims for healthcare providers to submit to medical insurance companies
- **Educator**. Trains medical insurance specialists
- **Editor**. Writes about health insurance
- **Consultant**. Provides billing and claim services to healthcare providers
- **Consumer claims assistant**. Files claims and appeals for low reimbursement on behalf of patients
- **Private billing**. Files claims for elderly and disabled patients

Qualifications for Medical Insurance Specialists

A medical insurance specialist must

- Understand medical terminology
- Have a basic knowledge of anatomy and physiology

- Have knowledge of conventions and rules used in diagnosis and procedures coding
- Have critical reading and comprehension skills
- Have basic math skills
- Have good oral and written communication skills
- Have the basic computer skills needed to enter and access data electronically
- Be ethical
- Be detail oriented

Medical Insurance Specialists Certification

The **American Health Information Association** (AHIMA) offers three certifications for medical insurance specialists. These are the **Certified Coding Specialists** (CCS), **the Certified Coding Specialists–Physician-Based** (CCS-P), and the **Certified Coding Associate** (CCA). Each certificate is awarded to medical insurance specialists who pass the corresponding examination.

The CCS covers surgery coding, inpatient documentation and data integrity, anatomy, physiology, and pharmacology. The CCS-P covers coding in physician-based settings such as physician offices, group practices, multispecialty clinics, and specialty centers. The medical insurance specialist reviews patient records and assigns numeric codes for each diagnosis and procedure. The CCA credential demonstrates coding competencies in both hospitals and physician practices. The CCA credential balances job experience with tested knowledge and is the first credential earned by new graduates.

The **American Academy of Professional Coders** (AAPC; aapc@aapcnatl .org) is another organization that offers two certifications. These are the **Certified Professional Coder** (CPC), focusing on physician offices and clinics, and the **Certified Professional Coder–Hospital** (CPC-H), which is designed for medical insurance specialists who work in hospitals.

Both AHIMA and AAPC award certificates to those who pass their corresponding certification examination.

CASE STUDY

CASE 1

An 83-year-old male patient talking to the medical billing specialist in his primary care practitioner's office about having to write a check for the co-pay and how Medicare and medical insurance has gotten too complicated. He was reminiscing about the 1950s, when going to the doctor was simpler. He then asks you the following questions. What is your best response?

QUESTION 1. Back in the 1950s, practically everyone had Blue Cross and Blue Shield. Everyone paid the same amount for the insurance. Why has that changed?
ANSWER: Blue Cross and Blue Shield uses a community-rate premium model where everyone pays the same premium regardless of their claims. Most medical insurers use an experienced-rate premium model where the premium is based on the claims submitted by the policyholder.

QUESTION 2. My son was recently laid off and has to buy his own health insurance. Why are individual health insurance policies more expensive than medical insurance provided by an employer?
ANSWER: A health insurance policy offered by an employer is a group policy where the premium is based on the claims submitted by all employees. The premium is relatively low if few employees are ill. Also, the employer typically pays a larger portion of the premium than the portion paid by the employee. The insured pays the entire premium for an individual policy and the premium may be based on the insured's health.

QUESTION 3. I heard that medical insurance companies must cover preexisting medical conditions. Why won't they do that any way?
ANSWER: An insurer establishes a premium based on certain risk and the probability that negative events will occur. For example, every 25-year-old man is exposed to similar risk such as injury related to working out or a car accident. Insurers use the probability that those events will occur within the group covered by the insurance policy. That is, a few 25-year-old men within the group covered by the insurance policy will experience those events—but most will not. However, preexisting conditions alter the probability factor. A person with a preexisting condition has a 100% chance of submitting many claims for reimbursements. Some insurers feel that the risk is too high—such as insuring a driver who has had frequent car accidents. Employers typically agree to higher premiums because the policy covers preexisting conditions. The cost of reimbursement is shared among all employees in the form of the premium.

QUESTION 4. Back in the 1950s we never had charity care. Everyone was able to see and pay their doctor. Shouldn't we do away with charity care?

ANSWER: In the 1950s, physicians practiced an informal form of charity care. It was common for a physician to set fees based on the patient's ability to pay. For example, a minimum fee might be charged to a low-income family. Under certain circumstances, the physician would tell the patient to pay when he could pay, knowing that the patient was unlikely to pay. However, a higher fee was charged to patients who could afford to pay. In essence, the higher fees offset the lower fees and the physician was able to care for all the patients and receive a desired income.

FINAL CHECKUP

1. **A revenue stream is**
   A. A product or service that is bought to bring in revenue.
   B. A product or service that is sold to bring in revenue.
   C. A product or service that is sold to pay premiums.
   D. None of the above.

2. **Payment by an insurer to a healthcare provider for a claim is called a**
   A. Premium.
   B. Reimbursement.
   C. Differential.
   D. Fee.

3. **Blue Cross**
   A. Provides surgery coverage
   B. Provides prescription medical coverage
   C. Provides physician medical coverage
   D. Provides hospital medical coverage

4. **The Social Security Act of 1965 created Medicare and Medicaid.**
   A. True
   B. False

5. **The experienced rating system sets a premium based on the experience of the person who is being insured.**
   A. True
   B. False

6. **Sick insurance was**

   A. An early version of medical insurance.
   B. Similar to disability insurance.
   C. Burial insurance.
   D. All of the above.

7. **Qualifications to receive Medicaid are uniform throughout the United States.**

   A. True
   B. False

8. **Medical insurers earn a profit by**

   A. Investing premiums.
   B. Denying claims.
   C. Extending the time between when the claim is filed and the claim is paid.
   D. All of the above.

9. **Blue Cross and Blue Shield set policy rates using the community-rating system.**

   A. True
   B. False

10. **Medicaid is a joint program operated by the federal and state governments to provide medical insurance for the indigent.**

    A. True
    B. False

CORRECT ANSWERS AND RATIONALES

1. B. A product or service that is sold to bring in revenue.
2. B. Reimbursement.
3. D. Provides hospital medical coverage.
4. A. True.
5. A. True.
6. B. Similar to disability insurance.
7. B. False.
8. D. All of the above.
9. A. True.
10. A. True.

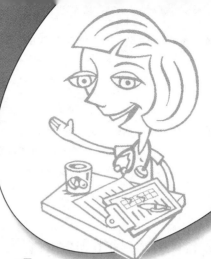

chapter 2

Ethical and Legal Aspects of Medical Billing

LEARNING OBJECTIVES

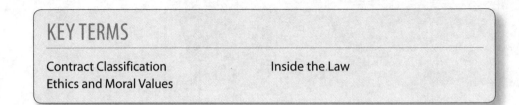

KEY TERMS

Contract Classification   Inside the Law
Ethics and Moral Values

1. Insight Into Medical Billing

"Did you know that Mrs. Roberts, the little, old, white-haired lady who was here this morning, is an alcoholic? Who would have thought?"

The medical insurance specialist mentioned this to the receptionist as they walked through the waiting room on their way to lunch. Just by chance a neighbor of Mrs. Roberts was waiting to be seen by the physician and had chatted with Mrs. Roberts before Mrs. Roberts left the office. She hadn't known that Mrs. Roberts was an alcoholic—until the medical insurance specialist told her and everyone in the waiting room.

What may at first appear to be innocent gossip can have far-reaching implications for medical insurance specialists and their employers because conversations regarding a patient are likely to reveal confidential medical information, which is a violation of medical ethics and the law.

After learning that her medical condition was told to everyone in the waiting room, Mrs. Roberts consulted an attorney who brought charges against the medical insurance specialist, the healthcare provider, and the healthcare facility. Furthermore, various government agencies were asked to investigate the medical record-keeping practices of the healthcare provider and of the healthcare facility.

Medical insurance specialists work with patients' confidential medical records and therefore must adhere to ethical and legal standards common to the medical profession. This chapter discusses those standards and how to comply with them.

2. Ethics and Medical Billing

Ethics is a standard of behavior that defines the right thing to do regardless of whether doing it is legal or illegal, convenient or inconvenient, rewarding or not. The standard might be defined by a professional association or by law, or by a more simple definition: the way everyone is expected to behave.

You have probably seen news stories about behaviors you felt were simply wrong, such as a former employer of a powerful elected official receiving a lucrative, no-bid, billion-dollar government contract. Your outrage was based on your ethics—not on the law. Some people may believe it is unethical for any government official to give a contract to a former employer, while others may disagree. Still other people will look the other way, saying, "It is unethical, but in this case we'll make an exception."

It is easy to be ethical if you're not personally involved. For example, many of us believe that everyone is entitled to the same medical care regardless of ability to pay for the care. Some people consider a healthcare provider who turns away a patient for financial reasons as being unethical.

Suppose you were the healthcare provider. A new patient arrives who has a long-term disease requiring many office and hospital visits. The patient is a Medicare client. Medicare reimburses you far less than private insurers do for the same procedures. This means you make less money treating a Medicare patient than you do treating a patient who has private medical insurance.

Should you tell this patient that you are no longer taking new patients? If you say no, then you're making an ethical decision that will lose you the opportunity to make more money from privately insured patients. If you say yes, then some people will consider you unethical because you turned away patients because they can't pay you as much as you want to earn.

Let's say you accept the patient for ethical reasons. The patient tells friends that he found a healthcare provider who is taking Medicare patients. Within a few days your office is filled with new patients, nearly all of whom are covered by Medicare.

Should you tell these patients that you are no longer taking new patients? If you say no, then you'll be losing substantial income because most of your time is spent performing procedures for low fees. Furthermore, you risk losing your non-Medicare patients who may experience longer wait times to get an appointment. If you say yes, then you'd be turning away patients because they couldn't pay your fee.

This is a tough question to answer, yet most healthcare providers must answer this question every day.

Ethics and Moral Values

Our standard of ethics stems from moral values that each of us forms based on conduct that our family, friends, neighbors, and religious and government leaders expect from us and what we expect from others. For many of us this means that we treat every person the way we want to be treated.

Would you want a medical insurance specialist to tell others that you are an alcoholic? Probably not. Then if you were the medical insurance specialist, would you tell a colleague that a patient is an alcoholic? At first you may say that you'll keep the patient's information confidential, but in reality all of us have a tendency to tell others gossip—"Don't tell anyone, but . . . ."

Gossiping probably doesn't violate moral values because many of us have grown up in a culture where it is expected that some rules will be broken. In fact, we tend to look strangely at anyone who always obeys the rulebook.

You have probably heard a football commentator saying that the referee should let the guys play the game and stop flagging them for every infraction of the rules. And you might ask a police officer to give you a break and not write a traffic ticket.

And it is not unusual to take a sick day even though you're not sick. Does this violate moral values? The rule states that sick days are to be used when you're sick. If you're not sick, then you should take a vacation day or personal day, but not a sick day.

Breaking the sick day rule is acceptable even if it shows that you're not totally truthful. In some cases you may give your supervisor a wink and a smile when saying that you're not feeling well and you might take a sick day tomorrow. Many supervisors "look the other way" and have a "Don't ask, don't tell" view of sick days. This holds true even if a local TV news camera crew interviews you on the beach while you are "sick."

Private corporations set their own rules, such as the sick day rule, and can penalize an employee for violating the rule. Termination is the worst penalty an employee can experience. However, government rules cannot be as easily overlooked. Violating a government rule can result in a fine and even imprisonment.

Suppose a government employee calls in sick when in reality she went to the beach. The employee committed fraud against the government—a serious crime. The employee accepted sick pay when in fact the employee wasn't sick. This is stealing money from the government.

There tends to be one set of moral values for violating rules created by the government and another set for violating rules that are created by relatives, friends, or our employer. That is, there is a higher ethical standard for certain rules than for other rules.

Medical insurance specialists and others in the healthcare profession follow rules created by the government, professional associations, and their employers. Government rules called *laws* must be followed. Rules created by professional associations and employers should be followed.

The medical insurance specialist who inadvertently told everyone in the waiting room that Mrs. Roberts is an alcoholic violated the law and ethics of the healthcare industry. Throughout this chapter you'll learn about laws that govern the healthcare industry and why you must have an unwavering degree of medical ethics when working in the healthcare field.

3. Legal Aspects of Medical Billing

Patients expect healthcare professionals to cure them, and when their expectations are not met, some patients take retribution by suing the healthcare provider and all those who were involved in their care.

Healthcare professionals are also targets of aggressive attorneys who seek patients who would otherwise not sue and convince them that they can recoup their losses by bringing legal action against those who provided them with healthcare.

Healthcare professionals are also watched by various government agencies to ensure that all laws and regulations that cover prescribing medication, record keeping, proper billing to Medicare and Medicaid, and a host of other aspects of healthcare are being followed.

Medical insurance specialists are exposed to potential legal action because they handle confidential patient information and prepare the bill and related documentation submitted to government agencies for payment. No one is immune to legal action, but you can minimize exposure to a lawsuit by knowing the law and regulations that govern the healthcare industry.

Inside the Law

A *law* is a rule that everyone must abide by. There are four classifications of law that you should know: common law, statutory law, administrative law, and case law.

Common law is a set of rules that comes about from common practice rather than a rule created by a governing body or by a government official. You probably have heard the term *common law marriage*. Two people who live together and act as if they are married for a reasonable period of time are considered married, just as if a judge, mayor, or minister married them. This is an example of common law.

Statutory law is a rule created by a legislative process. On the federal level, this is when the House of Representatives, the Senate, and the president of the United States agree on a rule. A similar process occurs on the state and local levels.

Administrative law is a rule enacted by a government official or a group of government officials in order to administer a statutory law. For example, statutory law created Medicare and Medicaid and granted authority for the administrative branch of government to appoint officials to run the Medicare and Medicaid programs. However, statutory law didn't contain all the fine regulations that are necessary to run Medicare and Medicaid. Administrative officials who run these programs create these regulations, which are known as administrative law.

Case law is a rule created by a court when interpreting statutory law and administrative law. The legislative process usually produces laws that are somewhat vague, such as Medicare will cover the hospitalization for the elderly. The term *hospitalization* is vague. It can mean a hospital stay for cancer treatment. It can also mean a hospital stay for a face-lift. Administrative law transforms vague terms into rules. That is, the administrator of Medicare may decide that hospitalization for a face-lift is not what Congress intended when it wrote the law. As a result, Medicare wouldn't cover hospital expenses for a face-lift.

However, a Medicare patient who receives a face-lift can challenge this rule in court. If the court agrees with the patient, then the court by its ruling creates case law that Medicare must cover hospitalization for a face-lift. Either party can usually appeal the decision to a higher court until it reaches the Supreme Court, whose decision is final. Case law is frequently referred to as legal precedents, which is usually followed by other courts as a rule of law.

Knowing all the laws that pertain to medical billing is a challenge. Fortunately, your healthcare facility's attorney can provide guidelines to follow that reflect the attorney's interpretation of common law, statutory law, administrative law, and case law that affect the healthcare professional. Healthcare facilities can also employ Compliance Officers who stay abreast of the guidelines effecting the administration of healthcare. These guidelines tell you what you can and cannot do.

Each day brings new administrative laws and case law that may change these guidelines. That is, yesterday you might have been permitted to look at all the information about a patient and tomorrow you may only be allowed to view a portion of that information. Therefore, it is important to review and adhere to the latest guidelines used by your healthcare facility. Following these guidelines lessens the chances that you and the healthcare facility will become involved in a legal action.

4. Civil Law

Civil law is a set of rules where the penalty is monetary. If you violate a civil law, a person whose rights you violated can take you to court seeking monetary damages to compensate them for the violation.

For example, Mrs. Roberts' rights were violated when the medical insurance specialist told people in the waiting room that she was an alcoholic. Mrs. Roberts can file civil charges in court seeking damages from the medical insurance specialist, the healthcare provider, and the healthcare facility. She must prove by a preponderance of evidence that her rights were violated and that the medical insurance specialist, the healthcare provider, and the healthcare facility violated her rights.

The medical insurance specialist, the healthcare provider, and the healthcare facility can defend themselves against the charges brought by Mrs. Roberts by going to court and challenging Mrs. Roberts' evidence and by providing their own evidence proving that Mrs. Roberts' rights were not violated or at least were not violated by the medical insurance specialist, the healthcare provider, or the healthcare facility.

Mrs. Roberts is called the **plaintiff**, and the medical insurance specialist, the healthcare provider, and the healthcare facility are the **defendants**.

The plaintiff and the defendants go to court and present their evidence to the judge and the jury. The jury listens to both sides and determines the facts. The jury is said to be the judge of facts. The judge also listens to both sides and interprets the law that the plaintiff claims the defendants violated. The **judge** is said to be the judge of law.

Suppose Mrs. Roberts claims that the defendants defamed her character, which is saying something about her that isn't true that hurts her reputation. She presents evidence such as witnesses to support her claim. The judge defines the facts that must be proven to support a charge of defamation of character for the jury based on the law. The **jury** decides if the evidence that Mrs. Roberts presented is fact and whether the facts support the claim of defamation of character.

If the jury decides in Mrs. Roberts' favor, then the defendants are guilty. However, no one goes to jail. Instead the jury, or sometimes the judge, answers two questions: (1) How much money should be awarded to Mrs. Roberts? (2) How much is each defendant responsible for the violation?

Answers to both questions must be based on a reasonable set of facts. That is, the jury can't simply pick an amount out of thin air or say one defendant is more responsible than the others because they picked his name out of a hat.

For example, the jury might base the award on the actual economic losses that Mrs. Roberts incurred, such as lost wages or medical expenses to treat emotional distress she endured because of the violation of her rights.

Determining how much each defendant is responsible for the injury is not an exact science. The jury might say that the medical insurance specialist is 10% at fault for making the statement in public. The healthcare facility might be 80% at fault for not properly training and supervising the medical insurance specialist. The healthcare provider might be 10% liable because he/she provided information about Mrs. Roberts to the medical insurance specialist.

You can think of these percentages as percentages of blame assessed to each defendant. The percentage is then applied to the monetary award to determine how much money each defendant must pay to Mrs. Roberts.

Nearly all healthcare workers and healthcare facilities are covered by malpractice insurance and liability insurance. The insurance company pays Mrs. Roberts nearly the entire award except for the deductible, which is paid by each defendant.

There are two types of awards: for compensatory damage and punitive damage. *Compensatory damage* is the real economic loss of the plaintiff such as lost wages and expenses. *Punitive damage* is a monetary value that punishes the defendant for violating the plaintiff's rights.

For example, the jury might award Mrs. Roberts $1,000 to compensate her for medical expenses related to emotional stress over the incident. The jury might also award her $25,000 in punitive damages to punish the defendant so that the defendant doesn't repeat the violation.

Civil court judges have wide latitude in some states to overrule the jury's verdict and award. Likewise, the plaintiff and the defendant have the right to appeal the verdict and the award to an appeals court. However, they must have a reason to appeal, such as the evidence didn't support the verdict or the judge improperly defined the law for the jury.

Many civil cases are settled before going to trial. A settlement is where the plaintiff and the defendant agree on the resolution of their differences. For example, the medical insurance specialist might apologize to Mrs. Roberts, and Mrs. Roberts might accept the apology without any monetary award. The defendant's insurance company may offer Mrs. Roberts money to drop the charges. If Mrs. Roberts accepts, then the case is closed and never goes to court.

There are many reasons plaintiffs and defendants settle a case. The insurance company might think the jury would award more than the money it proposes to give the plaintiff to settle the case. The plaintiff might accept the settlement thinking that the jury might award less than the offered amount.

Many times cases are settled without admitting guilt. That is, a defendant who is innocent settles the case for a fixed dollar amount rather than incur the expense of a trial and the risk of being found liable.

It is important to understand that a jury decides whether a defendant violated the plaintiff's rights based on the preponderance of the evidence—not whether the evidence proves the defendant is guilty beyond a reasonable doubt.

Let's say that the plaintiff brings a witness to court who testifies that she was in the room and heard the medical insurance specialist say that Mrs. Roberts is an alcoholic. The defendant doesn't call a witness to refute her claims. The jury believes that the witness's testimony is fact and therefore there is more evidence supporting the plaintiff's claim than there is evidence supporting the defendant's claim of innocence. The preponderance of the evidence supports the plaintiff.

In other words, a jury can find a defendant guilty if the plaintiff makes the defendant look guilty. The jury can return a guilty verdict even if it thinks that the defendant could be innocent.

5. Contracts

Civil law suits arise out of disputes over contracts or violation of a civil law. A *contract* is an agreement between two parties where one person agrees to do something and another agrees to give that person consideration for doing it. *Consideration* is usually money, but it can be anything of value, such as an automobile or house, or services such as someone fixing your car in exchange for you painting a room in his house.

A contract is a voluntary agreement between two people who are referred to as *a party to the contract*. A contract needs the following elements to be legally binding and enforced by the courts:

- There must be an offer to do something by one party.
- The offer must be communicated to the second party.
- The offer must be made in good faith—not as a joke.
- There must be an acceptance of the offer by the second party.
- The second party must accept the offer without duress—the party who makes the offer can't force the second party to accept the offer.
- The contract must define what both parties will do.
- There must be a date reflecting when the parties agreed to the contract.
- There must be a termination date after which neither party is bound by the terms of the contract.
- There must be consideration.
- The offer must be legal. That is, a bet placed with a bookmaker is not a legal contract because gambling in an unlicensed facility is illegal.
- Both parties to the contract must be mentally competent to enter into the contract. For example, someone who is a minor couldn't enter into a

contract for medical care because he or she lacks the legal stature. A minor is a person who is younger than 18 years in most states. In some states, a minor is a person who is younger than 21 years. A parent or legal guardian can enter into a contract on behalf of a minor. However, medical care—sufficient to save the minor's life—can be given to a minor in an emergency without permission from a parent or legal guardian.

If an agreement does not conform to the legal definition of a contract, then the agreement is *voided*. That is, the courts cannot enforce the terms of the contract. However, an agreement that fulfills the legal definition of a contract except that one party is incompetent is a *voidable contract*.

Voidable means that the party who is incompetent has the choice to void (ignore) the contract or enforce the contract. The party who is competent cannot void the contract. Suppose a 17-year-old, who appears to be 21, signs a contract to purchase an automobile at a great price. The 17-year-old can back out of the contract by claiming she is incompetent to enter into a contract.

Since only one party of the contract is incompetent, the contract is voidable and not void. The party selling the car can't say, "I just learned that you are only 17 years old, so I'm not going to sell you the car."

The 17-year-old can say, "I'm 17 years old and therefore legally incompetent, so I'm not going to buy your car." Alternatively, the 17-year-old can say, "I'm 17 years old and legally incompetent; however, my parent is authorized to enter the contract on my behalf. Therefore, I'm buying your car even if you no longer want to sell it to me because I'm incompetent."

In simple terms, the party who is competent doesn't have the option to void a signed contract. The party who is incompetent has the option to either void the contract or enforce the contract.

Contract Classification

There are two classifications of contracts: implied contract and express contract.

An *implied contract* is an agreement two parties enter into by their actions or inactions. Nothing is in writing and there is no verbal agreement. Implied contracts are frequently entered into in an emergency room when an unconscious patient arrives for treatment. It is implied that the patient agrees to treatment and assumes the responsibility to pay for the treatment.

Another implied contract occurs when a healthcare provider prepares an injection and the patient rolls up his sleeve to receive the injection. Neither party stated contract terms nor agreed to the contract verbally or in writing. However, their actions implied the offer (preparing the injection) and an acceptance (rolling up the sleeve). The date of the contract is the current date, as is the termination date. Consideration is the standard fee for the injection.

An *express contract* is either a verbal or written agreement where the terms are openly stated. A verbal express contract is where the components of a contract are expressed in words such as buying groceries. A written express contract is where the components of the contract are written and signed by both parties.

Regardless of the classification of the contract, if one person does not fulfill a term of the contract, then there is a *breach of contract* and the other person can ask the civil court to enforce the contract by requiring the other person to abide by the terms of the contract.

6. Types of Civil Law

Violation of a civil law is called a tort. A *tort* is a civil wrong made against a person or property. A tort can be unintentional or intentional.

An *unintentional tort* is where a person did not mean to cause injury to another person, which is the case involving the medical insurance specialist who didn't intend for the conversation to be heard by anyone but the receptionist.

An *intentional tort* is where a person intended to cause injury to another person. The medical insurance specialist would have committed an intentional tort by going into the waiting room, asking for everyone to be quiet, and announcing that Mrs. Roberts is an alcoholic.

Healthcare providers are more likely to commit unintentional torts because their actions are usually not intentional, but they might be negligent. *Negligence* is a tort that occurs when a person performs an action or causes an action to be performed by another person that is unreasonable or is made without regard for the consequences of the action. Negligence is also committed when a person fails to exercise ordinary care and as a result injures a patient.

For example, a healthcare provider who mistakenly punctures a blood vessel during surgery is negligent by his or her action. Likewise, a healthcare provider is negligent by inaction if the healthcare provider doesn't stop a patient from bleeding.

It is important to understand that a poor outcome of a procedure or treatment is not necessarily negligence. Some undesired outcomes could occur even when a procedure or treatment is performed to the normal standard of care.

Medical procedures and treatments have some degree of risk that both the patient and the healthcare provider agree to take. The healthcare provider isn't negligent if a potential risk is realized as long as the healthcare provider has used the care any reasonable healthcare provider would give when performing the procedure or giving treatment.

Malpractice is a tort that occurs when a person who has special knowledge and training provides care that does not conform to professional standards and that care injures a patient. For example, an angiogram is a procedure where dye is injected into a patient to expose blood vessels on an X-ray. Some patients are allergic to the dye. A healthcare provider is guilty of malpractice if he or she doesn't determine the patient's allergies before performing the angiogram.

Negligence and malpractice are similar, but different. The key differences are skills and training. The jury uses the reasonable person rule to determine negligence. That is, would a reasonable person in the position of the defendant perform the same action? If so, then the defendant is not negligent. If not, then the person is negligent.

In a malpractice case, the jury must determine whether the defendant had the necessary skills and training to perform the action and whether the action was performed according to widely acceptable practice. If so, then the defendant is not guilty of malpractice. If the defendant has the skills and training and the defendant's action was not in accordance with acceptable practice, then the defendant is guilty of malpractice.

An expert witness usually testifies in malpractice cases to define a widely acceptable practice. The expert witness basically tells the jury how the procedure should be performed.

In contrast, jurors may use their own experience to define the action a reasonable person would have taken in the situation experienced by the person charged with negligence. A medical insurance specialist can be exposed to charges of negligence but rarely malpractice. Healthcare providers are exposed to malpractice charges rather than negligence because they provide patients with professional care.

Malpractice cases usually are governed by the doctrine of res ipsa loquitur, which determines the evidence a plaintiff may present to prove that the defendant committed malpractice. The doctrine of res ipsa loquitur basically means that the events speak for it. That is,

- The action that caused the injury to the plaintiff would not have occurred in the normal course of events if the healthcare provider had used reasonable care.

- The healthcare provider had exclusive control over the cause of the injury to the plaintiff.
- The plaintiff did not contribute to the action.

For example, a patient who had undergone gallbladder surgery last year is now complaining about nausea and vomiting. Her condition has been getting worse over the past 2 weeks. The healthcare provider noticed a strange object on the patient's X-ray, so a surgeon was called in to perform exploratory surgery to further identify the object. The object was a towel that had eroded. The surgeon could make out the name of the hospital on the towel. This was enough evidence to enable the patient to enforce the res ipsa loquitur doctrine to prove that the surgeon who removed the gallbladder was negligent.

Here's why:

- The towel would not have been left inside the patient if the surgeon had used reasonable care.
- The surgeon had exclusive control over the gallbladder surgery.
- The patient did not do anything to cause the towel to be left inside her body.

7. The Feasances

Healthcare providers are also exposed to three other types of torts. These are malfeasance, misfeasance, and nonfeasance. **Feasance** means the performance of an act. Therefore, these torts relate to the performance of the healthcare provider.

- **Malfeasance** occurs when the healthcare provider performs a totally wrongful and unlawful act such as the medical receptionist giving a patient the wrong medication without any direction from a healthcare provider. A medical receptionist cannot dispense medication (unlawful act) and the wrong medication was given to the patient (totally wrongful act).
- **Misfeasance** occurs when a lawful act is performed in an illegal or improper manner. This happens when a healthcare provider doesn't use a sterile technique when changing a dressing on a patient. The healthcare provider can legally change the dressing (lawful act), but doesn't use the correct technique (improper manner).
- **Nonfeasance** occurs when a lawful act was not performed when it should have been performed. For example, a healthcare provider recognizes symptoms of appendicitis but instead of asking for a test or calling a surgeon, the healthcare provider sends the patient home (not performed).

8. The Four Ds of Negligence

There are four elements that must be presented before a healthcare provider is guilty of negligence. These are

- **Duty**. The healthcare provider owes a duty to the patient. A primary physician owes a duty to tell a patient that the mole on his face might be cancerous. However, a physician who casually meets a person on the train and notices the mole doesn't have a duty to tell the person that the mole might be cancerous.

- **Dereliction**. The healthcare provider breaches the duty. That is, the primary physician notices the mole but doesn't do anything about it.

- **Direct cause**. The breach of duty injured the patient. For example, the cancer on the patient's face spread into the nose.

- **Damages**. The patient is entitled to damages from the healthcare provider.

Some states have imposed laws that restrict claims brought against healthcare providers in order to reduce frivolous lawsuits. For example, a medical review panel composed of physicians and a neutral attorney may examine the facts about the claim to be assured that the facts support the claim. If so, then the case goes to court; otherwise the charges are dismissed.

Physicians are vicariously liable for actions of their employees on the job under the respondeat superior doctrine, which means "let the master answer." An employee while on the job is an agent of the physician. An agent is someone who performs an action on behalf of another person. This means that the physician is vicariously liable for the action of the medical insurance specialist if those actions occur within the scope of the job.

For example, the physician who employed the medical insurance specialist is vicariously liable to Mrs. Roberts by the medical insurance specialist's action of revealing Mrs. Roberts' patient information.

In order to prove vicarious liability

- An **agency** must exist between the employer and the person who commits the action such as the physician who employed the medical insurance specialist.

- The **action** must have occurred within the scope of the employee's job. The medical insurance specialist was working at the time that the patient information was revealed and the patient information was obtained as part of the medical insurance specialist's job.

Regardless of the intent, the medical insurance specialist's action is a tort. The nature of the tort depends on the type of law that was violated. Here are common torts that a medical insurance specialist must understand.

- **Invasion of privacy**. A person intrudes into the private affairs of another without permission.

- **Defamation of character**. A person causes the publication of a false statement that damages another person's reputation.

- **Malice**. A person causes the publication of a false statement that damages another person's reputation and knows that the statement is false before the statement is published.

- **Slander**. A false statement is said in the presence of another person.

- **Libel**. A false statement made in writing.

- **Informed consent**. A person agrees to allow something to happen such as permitting the healthcare professional to share the person's medical records with the person's insurance company.

- **Standards of care**. Legal guidelines that specify the level of care a patient must receive from a healthcare provider.

- **Malfeasance**. A healthcare provider has a duty to do something but doesn't. The healthcare provider's lack of action results in an injury of another person.

9. Types of Criminal Law

Criminal law is a set of rules that provides for fines and/or incarceration if the rules are violated. It is categorized by the type of penalty that can be imposed if the law is violated. These categories are felony, misdemeanor, and disorderly person.

- **Felony**. A felony is a serious crime such as murder. A person who is convicted of a felony is likely to be imprisoned.

- **Misdemeanor**. A misdemeanor is a lesser crime such as an assault. A person convicted of a misdemeanor is likely to receive an alternative sentence that does include incarceration.

- **Disorderly person**. A disorderly person is a minor crime such as causing a disturbance that usually results in a fine.

Healthcare professionals are exposed to violations of criminal law. Some of the more common criminal laws they are exposed to are

- **Fraud**. This is an intentional deception that results in an injury to another person and can occur when a healthcare provider or healthcare facility intentionally submits false medical bills to Medicare, Medicaid, or medical insurance companies.

- **Battery**. This is the intentional touching of a person without the patient's consent such as when a medical procedure is performed on a patient without the patient's consent.

- **Assault**. This is the intentional threat to bring about harm to a person such as pointing a hypodermic syringe at a patient. Although medication in the syringe helps the patient, the patient is harmed when the medication is injected into the patient. Healthcare professionals avoid assault and battery changes by having the patient sign a consent form before the patient is seen by the healthcare professional or before a procedure is performed on the patient.

- **False imprisonment**. This is the intentional and unlawful restraint or confinement of a person by another person. Restraints include side rails on hospital beds. Raising all four side rails prevents the patient from getting out of bed, which is unlawful and therefore false imprisonment. The refusal to release a patient from a healthcare facility is also false imprisonment.

10. Confidentiality

In 1996, Congress passed the **Health Insurance Portability and Accountability Act** (HIPAA) that established standards for securing patients' health information and required the healthcare industry to maintain privacy and confidentiality of any health information that identifies a patient. This includes the transfer of health information electronically, health information written on paper, and health information that is discussed among healthcare providers.

The medical insurance specialist who told the receptionist—and patients in the waiting room—that Mrs. Roberts is an alcoholic violated HIPPA because Mrs. Roberts' healthcare information wasn't kept private and confidential.

A patient must give written consent to the healthcare provider before the healthcare provider can share the patient's medical information with anyone. This includes sharing medical information with the nurse who is providing healthcare to the patient.

HIPAA requires that only necessary health information about a patient be shared with others who need to know the information. This restriction also applies to hospital administrators, the accounting department, attorneys, insurance companies, and anyone else who seeks information about the patient.

For example, a hospital medical laboratory technician testing Mrs. Roberts' blood doesn't need to know Mrs. Roberts' name and address. All that is necessary is Mrs. Roberts' patient identification number and maybe her initials and room number.

The healthcare facility must establish clear policies and procedures on how patient's medical information is shared. Furthermore, a written contract must be signed by business associates, such as attorneys, clearly stating the business associate is obligated to maintain patient confidentiality.

Failure to abide by HIPAA exposes the healthcare professional and the healthcare facility to legal action by both the patient and the federal government.

As a medical insurance specialist, you are privy to patients' medical information and therefore are at risk of violating HIPAA. You can avoid violating HIPAA by staying within the following guidelines:

- Don't disclose patient information even to a colleague unless there is a need for the person to access this information.
- Make sure the patient has signed a written consent authorizing you to share patient information with another person.
- Treat all patient information as confidential even if the information appears to be general information about the patient.
- Don't assume that the patient won't mind you sharing patient information with another person.
- Ensure that you convey authorized patient information to another person in private and not in the hallway or in an area where your conversation can be overheard.
- Position the computer screen so that only you can see patient information that appears on the screen.
- Remove patient information immediately from fax machines, copiers, and printers. If you print patient information, then immediately pick up the information at the printer.
- Don't use the patient's name when discussing patient information with a colleague because others might overhear your conversation.

- Provide the minimum amount of information when leaving a message for a patient. Simply say, "Please call Dr. Tom's office." Don't say, "Please call Dr. Tom's office regarding the bill for your blood test."

- File all patient information immediately after you have finished reading it.

- Don't leave patient information in plain view or on a desk.

- Conceal patient information if someone walks over to your desk.

- A patient's medical information cannot be released without written consent from a patient except when the medical information is subpoenaed. A subpoena is an order of the court that can be issued by a judge or an attorney. This means you cannot release patient information to a law enforcement officer unless the officer presents you with a subpoena.

- You don't have the right to disregard HIPAA regardless of the circumstance.

- Don't assume that a patient has signed a consent form allowing you to share the patient's health information with another person. Always determine if the signed consent form is on file.

CASE STUDY

CASE 1

A 46-year-old woman who owns and manages small business arrives at her practitioner's office. She speaks with the medical billing specialist questioning the billing practices of the practitioner. Repeatedly, she points out that she knows the rules of how a business is run and how those rules can be bent especially to cut down the "red tape" and save money for both the business and the customer. She asks you the following questions. What is the best response?

QUESTION 1. My co-pay is minuscule compared with what the practitioner receives from my health insurance company. Can't we pretend I paid the co-pay?
ANSWER: The co-pay is small compared with the reimbursement by the insurer; however, the co-pay cannot be waived because that could be perceived as insurance fraud. You have a contract with the insurer that states you will pay the practitioner $30 per visit and the insurer will reimburse the practitioner for the reasonable and customary fee that exceeds the co-pay. Likewise, the practitioner has a contract with the insurer that states all except $30 of the reasonable and customary fee will be paid by the insurer. If the practitioner did not collect the

co-pay, then the reimbursement by the insurer could be considered 100% of the fee, which violates both contracts with the insurer.

QUESTION 2. A 32-year-old woman made an appointment to see the practitioner. She is not the practitioner's patient and is seeing the practitioner for the first time. She presents her insurance identification to the medical billing specialist when she walks into the waiting room. The medical billing specialist tells her that the practitioner does not have an arrangement with her insurer and therefore she must pay cash for the visit. She becomes indignant and threatens to sue the practitioner if anything happens to her because the practitioner didn't see her and she leaves the office. Would she be successful suing the practitioner?
ANSWER: Unlikely. The practitioner has a duty to the practitioner's patients; however, she is not the practitioner's patient, therefore there is no dereliction of duty. The patient needs to prove that the dereliction of duty was the direct cause of damage to her. She appeared stable, alert, oriented, and able to care for herself, so there is no apparent injury.

QUESTION 3. A patient complained to the practitioner that the office staff, including the medical billing specialist, disregarded the privacy of patients including her. She said that while sitting in the waiting room she could hear the staff talking among themselves and with patients at the desk about patients' medical conditions and test results. Furthermore, she reported that she heard another practitioner explain to a patient the importance of adhering to treatment for his diabetes. Was the patient correct?
ANSWER: Yes. The Health Insurance Portability and Accountability Act (HIPAA) mandates that all persons who have access to healthcare information maintain patient confidentiality. It is not unusual that staff is not aware that conversation within the office can be easily heard by patients sitting in the waiting room. Many times those conversations contain patient information.

QUESTION 4. The last patient of the day is a sweet elderly lady. Nearly all the office staff has left except for the medical billing specialist. She walks to the reception desk and tells the medical billing specialist that she left the sample of medication that the practitioner gave her in the examination room. She asks the medical specialist to retrieve the sample. What should the medical specialist do?
ANSWER: The medical billing specialist should relay the message to the practitioner then follow the practitioner's instructions. Even if the medical specialist knows that the elderly patient is truthful and sees the sample medication in the examination room, the medical billing specialist is not allowed to give a package of medication to the patient without direct instructions from the practitioner; otherwise, this may be considered malfeasance.

FINAL CHECKUP

1. **A contract can be**

   A. Written
   B. Verbal
   C. Created by the actions of two people
   D. All of the above

2. **A healthcare provider who performs a totally wrongful and unlawful act commits**

   A. Misfeasance
   B. Malfeasance
   C. Nonfeasance
   D. None of the above

3. **A healthcare provider who does not perform a lawful act when it should have been performed commits**

   A. Misfeasance
   B. Malfeasance
   C. Nonfeasance
   D. None of the above

4. **All contracts are voidable.**

   A. True
   B. False

5. **The promise to do something for consideration in a contract is called an offer.**

   A. True
   B. False

6. **An average person who fails to exercise ordinary care commits**

   A. Malpractice
   B. Negligence
   C. Feasence
   D. All of the above

7. **A physician can be held liable for his or her employee's actions because an agency exists.**

   A. True
   B. False

8. **Consideration in a contract is**

    A. Money

    B. Performance of an action

    C. A house

    D. All of the above

9. **Case law is a rule created by a court when interpreting statutory law and administrative law.**

    A. True

    B. False

10. **The courts must create all terms of a contract.**

    A. True

    B. False

CORRECT ANSWERS AND RATIONALES

1. D. All of the above
2. D. None of the above
3. B. Malfeasance
4. B. False
5. A. True
6. B. Negligence
7. A. True
8. D. All of the above
9. A. True
10. B. False

chapter 3

Medical Terminology and Procedures

LEARNING OBJECTIVES

1. Insight Into Medical Terminology and Procedures
2. The Secret to Understanding Medical Language
3. Mastering Medical Terminology
4. Medical Tests, Procedures, and Treatments

KEY TERMS

Strategy for Learning Medical
Terminology

1. Insight Into Medical Terminology and Procedures

Get an ABG, CBC, Chem 7, type and cross. Give him adenosine six milligrams IV push. Stat.

Sounds like an opening scene from a medical television program where a practitioner barks orders to the medical team as it swings into full gear to save a patient's life.

IV and stat are words you know, but since the other medical terminology isn't in your daily vocabulary—at least not yet—you probably wouldn't have a clue of what the physician is asking the medical team to do.

The practitioner in this example is telling the medical team to withdraw blood from the patient (ABG means arterial blood gas) and send the blood to the laboratory for testing (CBC means complete blood count and Chem 7 is a set of blood tests). The results of these tests give clues as to what might be wrong with the patient. The physician is also asking the medical team to identify the patient's blood type (type and cross) in case the patient needs a transfusion. And the medical team is asked to give the patient the drug adenosine (adenosine 6 mg) directly into the patient's intravenous (IV push) to stabilize the patient's irregular heartbeat—and all this happens immediately (stat).

As a medical insurance specialist you'll need to become fluent in medical terminology in order to properly code medical procedures to prepare medical bills for a healthcare facility. Learning medical terminology might seem overwhelming at first. However, in this chapter you'll learn the secret that will make understanding medical technology easy for you.

2. The Secret to Understanding Medical Language

The secret to understanding the meaning of a medical word is in the word itself. This might sound a bit like hocus-pocus, but no magic is involved.

Here's a test. What is myocarditis? You don't need to look up this term in a medical dictionary if you do a little dissection:

- **Prefix**. The beginning part of a word that qualifies the meaning of the word such as *pre* in preschool. *Pre* means "before." Prefixes may also indicate a number, time, or location.

- **Combining form**. That's a root ending with a vowel. It helps with pronunciation when adding suffixes that begin with a consonant.

- **Root**. The central part of a word (Table 3–1). The root in preschool is school.

- **Suffix**. The end part of a word that changes the meaning of the word. In the word hopeless, the root is *hope* and the suffix is *less,* which reverses the meaning of hope. It can also refer to a condition, procedure, disease, or disorder.

Medical terms are built using a prefix, root, suffix, and combining forms so that the term itself defines the word. Let's see how this works by dissecting **myocarditis** into its parts. *Myo* means "muscle," *cardio* refers to the "heart,"

TABLE 3–1 Root Words for Major Parts of the Body

Organ	Root	Organ	Root
Mouth	Stomato	Liver	Hepta
Teeth	Dento	Kidney	Nephro or ene
Tongue	Glosso/linguo	Testis	Orchido
Gums	Gingiv	Ovary	Oophoro
Brain	Encephalo	Uterus	Hystero or metro
Stomach	Gastro	Uterine tubes	Salpingo
Intestine	Entero	Skin	Dermo
Large intestine	Colo	Breast	Masto/mammo
Anus/rectum	Procoto	Bones	Osteo
Bladder	Cysto	Heart	Cardio
Veins	Phlebo or veno	Nose	Rhino
Blood	Hemo or emia	Lungs	Pneumo or pulmo

and *itis* is the suffix meaning "inflammation." Let's assemble the definitions to learn the meaning of myocarditis.

- **Muscle heart inflammation**. "Heart inflammation" makes sense. *Myocarditis* is an inflammation of the heart. However, "muscle" is probably a little confusing. You know the heart is a muscle, but that's not what myo refers to when speaking about the heart. You'll need a little anatomy to understand this part. The heart has three layers. Myo refers to the middle of the three layers. We can then rephrase the definition this way: Inflammation of the heart muscle.

Suppose we want to say that the outer layer of the heart is inflamed. The prefix *peri* means "around." All we need to do is replace the prefix *myo* with the prefix *peri*.

- **Pericarditis**. This means an inflammation of the layer around the heart.

The prefix *endo* is used to refer to "inner." Therefore, inflammation of the inner layer of the heart is *endocarditis*.

A prefix is independent of the root. This means *endo* always refers to "inner"—not just the inner layer of the heart. Likewise, *peri* always means around—around whatever the root is. And the root *myo* always refers to muscle and not only the muscle layer of the heart.

A suffix works similarly. The suffix *itis* refers to the inflammation of something—not just inflammation of the heart.

3. Mastering Medical Terminology

Now that you've learned the secret behind understanding medical terminology (prefix, root, suffix), it's time to focus on learning prefixes, roots, and suffixes that are commonly used in medical billing and coding.

Each major part of the body is identified by one or more root words. These words are derived from Greek or Latin words that describe the body parts. Table 3–1 lists parts of the body and its corresponding root word that you'll see used when billing and coding procedures are performed on those parts of the body. You'll find a complete list of root words at the following Web site: www.dmu.edu/medterms/basics.

Table 3–2 contains commonly used prefixes that you'll need to learn in order to properly handle billing and coding for the medical provider. Remember that a prefix is placed at the beginning of a root word to modify the meaning of the root word.

TABLE 3–2 Commonly Used Prefixes	
Prefix	**Meaning**
Mega-	Large
A-, An-	Without, away from, negative, not
Ante-	Before, toward
Anti-	Against, counter
Brady-	Slow
Dys-	Bad, difficult, painful
End-, Endo-,	Within, in, inside
Hemi-	Half
Hyper-	Excessive, increased
Hypo-	Deficient, decreased
Inter-	Between, among
Intra-	Within, inside
Micro	Small
Macro	Large
Neo-	New, strange
Per-	Excessive, through
Peri-	Surrounding, around
Poly-	Many
Post-	After
Pre-	Before
Sub-	Below
Super-, Supra-	Above, excessive
Tachy-	Fast, rapid

Table 3–3 lists commonly used suffixes. Remember that a suffix is placed at the end of the root word to change or further describe the root word. You should become familiar with these suffixes.

Strategy for Learning Medical Terminology

Prefixes, root words, and suffixes seem strange at first because they are not part of your working vocabulary. However, they can easily become part of your working vocabulary if you develop a plan for learning them.

TABLE 3–3   Commonly Used Suffixes in Medical Terminology

Suffix	Definition
-itis	Inflammation
-osis	Abnormal condition
-ectomy	Remove
-otomy	To cut into
-ostomy	To make an opening
A or an	Without, none
-megaly	Enlarged
-scopy/-scopic	To look, observe
-graphy/-graph	Recording an image
-gram	The image
-ology/-ologist	Study, specialize in
-algia	Pain

If you're overwhelmed right now by the thought of having to memorize a seemingly endless amount of medical words, stop. Take a time out. You are in good company because medical students, physicians, nurses, and others in the medical profession felt the same way when they were learning medical terminology. Each of them developed a strategy for learning these words.

Here's a winning strategy that you can use to learn medical terminology. Learn three prefixes, roots, and suffixes every 2 or 3 days. We call them the prefixes, roots, and suffixes of the day. Don't try to learn all the prefixes, roots, and suffixes at the same time because you'll experience an information overload.

Start by learning roots of common parts of the body, such as the heart and lungs, because you'll find it easy to associate the root (cardio) with the part of the body (heart) that you already know.

Associate suffix (itis) with a condition (inflammation). This too would be easy to do because you already know many of the conditions.

And then associate prefixes (neo) with its meaning (new). You already know the meaning of many prefixes.

Find the prefixes, root words, and suffixes of the day in articles and advertisements on popular medical Web sites such as www.webmd.com. When you see them, stop a moment and dissect the word into its prefix, root word, and suffix and then see if you can derive the meaning of the word from its components.

Do this for several weeks and you'll be surprised how quickly medical terminology becomes part of your working vocabulary.

4. Medical Tests, Procedures, and Treatments

Insurers reimburse healthcare providers according to the test, procedure, or treatment that the healthcare provider performs on the patient. A *test* is an examination that measures something. A *procedure* is a course of action that achieves a result. And a *treatment* is a type of procedure that relieves illness or injury.

When a patient goes to a physician feeling ill, the physician assesses the patient—top to bottom—looking for signs and symptoms of the problem. A *sign* is something that is abnormal such as a lump in the patient's armpit. A *symptom* is a problem reported to the practitioner by the patient. The practitioner must decide if the sign—and other signs—is a symptom of a condition or is of no significance.

Let's say that a patient has a lump in his armpit with other signs such as sudden weight loss and disruption of normal bowel movements. The patient's report of the lump is a symptom. Sudden weight loss and difficulty with bowel movements are signs. Collectively these signs and symptoms might be cancer.

After assessing the patient, the practitioner may need a medical test to verify the suspicion that the patient has a particular condition. In this example, the practitioner probably wants a pathologist to conduct a microscopic examination of the lump to determine whether the lump is cancerous. A *pathologist* is a physician who identifies diseased tissues.

A biopsy (procedure) is performed to remove a tissue sample of the lump so the pathologist can examine (test) the sample. If the pathologist diagnoses that the lump is cancerous, then the practitioner orders that the patient receive chemotherapy (treatment). In this case, the medical insurance specialist prepares bills for the practitioner's assessment, the biopsy procedure, the microscopic examination, and the chemotherapy treatment.

There are numerous tests, procedures, and treatments that are performed, and it is critical for you to be familiar with the more common of them so you can properly bill insurers. Table 3–4 contains the more common tests, Table 3–5 lists the most frequently performed medical procedures, and Table 3–6 shows treatments that you are likely to encounter each day.

TABLE 3–4 A List of Common Medical Tests

Medical Test	Description
Abdominal ultrasound	Examines abdominal organs using sound waves
ACTHs stimulation test	Diagnoses endocrine disorders
Amniocentesis	Sample of the amniotic fluid surrounding a fetus
Angiography	X-ray blood vessels
Arteriography	X-ray arteries
Barium enema	Shows the image of the lower gastrointestinal tract on an X-ray
Barium swallow	Shows the image of the upper gastrointestinal tract on an X-ray
Bone density scan	X-ray scan used to measure the density of your bones
Bone scan	Creates images of bones on a computer screen or on film
Bronchoscopy	Flexible tube with a small light and camera to examine the airways of the lung
Capsule endoscopy	Swallowable capsule containing a tiny camera takes pictures of the GI tract
Cardiac catheterization	Explores coronary arteries using a fine tube
Chorionic villus sampling	Test used during pregnancy to diagnose birth defects
Colposcopy	Examination of the vagina and cervix to determine the cause of an abnormal Pap smear
Complete blood count	Determines the number of red blood cells, white blood cells, and platelets in a sample of blood
Computed axial tomography (CAT) scan	A series of detailed pictures of inside the body created by a computer linked to an X-ray machine
Coronary angiography	The heart and blood vessels are filmed while the heart pumps showing problems such as a blockage caused by atherosclerosis

(Continued)

TABLE 3–4 A List of Common Medical Tests *(Continued)*	
Medical Test	**Description**
EKG, ECG	Electrocardiogram (ECG or EKG) is a graphic record of the electrical activity of the heart
Echocardiography	Uses ultrasonic waves to record the heart's position, motion of the walls, or internal parts such as the valves
Esophagogastroduodenoscopy (EGD)	Endoscope examination of the lining of the esophagus, stomach, and upper duodendum to diagnose cancer or other abnormalities
Electroencephalogram	Recording of the brain's electrical activity
Electromyography (EMG)	Measures the response of muscle fibers to electrical activity
Electron beam computed tomography (EBCT)	Identifies and measures calcium buildup in and around the coronary arteries
Electronystagmogram (ENG)	Test the vestibular system to help diagnose balance problems
Endoscopic ultrasound	Uses an endoscope and sound waves to create a sonogram of internal tissues and organs
Esophagoscopy	Examines the esophagus using a lighted tube to diagnose cancer, gastroesophageal reflux disease (GERD) and other conditions
Esophagogastroduodenoscopy (EGD)	Uses an endocsope to examine the lining of the esophagus, stomach, and upper duodendum to diagnose cancer or other abnormalities of the esophagus, stomach, and duodendum
Esophagram	X-rays of the esophagus
Fecal occult blood test	Checks for blood in stool
Fluoroscopy	X-ray
Functional magnetic resonance imaging (fMRI)	Used to observe functioning in the brain by detecting changes in chemical composition, blood flow, or both

(Continued)

TABLE 3–4   A List of Common Medical Tests *(Continued)*

Medical Test	Description
Gastroscopy	Examines the upper intestinal tract using a flexible tube
Genetic testing	Uses DNA to identify a genetic alteration
Hysterosalpingography	X-ray of the uterus and fallopian tubes
Intravenous pyelography (IVP)	X-ray study of the kidneys, ureters, and bladder
Laryngoscopy	Examination of the larynx
Lipoprotein profile	Measures cholesterol
Lower GI series	X-rays the large intestine, which includes the colon and rectum
Lymphangiography	X-ray of the lymphatic system
Mediastinoscopy	A tube is inserted into the chest to view organs between the lymph nodes and the lungs
MRI Magnetic resonance imaging	Creates detailed pictures inside the body using magnetic fields linked to a computer
Myelogram	X-ray examination used to detect abnormalities of the spine, spinal cord, or surrounding structures
Nephrotomogram	X-rays of the kidneys
NMRI Nuclear magnetic resonance imaging	Magnet linked to a computer creates images of inside the body
Nuclear medicine scan	Small amounts of radioactive material is used to create an image of inside the body
Pap test	Cells collected from the cervix for examination under a microscope
Pelvic laparoscopy celioscopy	Examines and treat abdominal and pelvic organs
Percutaneous transhepatic cholangiography	X-ray the hepatic and common bile ducts
Positron emission tomography (PET) scan	Computerized image of the metabolic activity of body tissues
Proctosigmoidoscopy	Uses a sigmoidoscope to examine the rectum and the lower part of the colon

(Continued)

TABLE 3–4 A List of Common Medical Tests (*Continued*)	
Medical Test	**Description**
Proton magnetic resonance spectroscopic imaging	Uses magnetic resonance imaging (MRI) to measure activity at the cellular level
Radionuclide scanning	Small amount of radioactive material are used to scan internal body parts
Sigmoidoscopy	Inspection of the lower colon using a sigmoidoscope
Sonogram ultrasound	A computer picture of inside the body created using sound waves
Stereotactic biopsy	Uses a computer and a three-dimensional scanning device to find a tumor site and remove tissue for examination under a microscope
Stress test	Records the heartbeat, breathing rate, and blood pressure during exercise
Tilt table test	Used to diagnose patients with unexplained fainting spells
Tomography	Creates pictures inside of body using a computer X-ray machine
Transabdominal ultrasound	Examines the organs in the abdomen using an ultrasound device
Transrectal ultrasound	Examines the prostate with ultrasound device
Transvaginal ultrasound	Ultrasound device used to examine the vagina
Ultrasound test	Ultrasound device used to examine the body
Upper GI series	A series of X-rays of the upper digestive system
Voiding cystourethrogram	X-ray examination of the bladder and lower urinary tract
Xeroradiography	X-ray in which pictures are recorded on paper
X-ray	Used to diagnose diseases by making pictures of the inside of the body

TABLE 3–5 Commonly Seen Procedures in Medical Billing	
Procedure	Description
Biopsy	Removal of cells or tissues for examination under a microscope
Bone marrow biopsy	Removal of a tissue sample from the bone marrow with a needle for examination under a microscope
Chamberlain procedure	A tube is inserted into the chest to view the tissues and organs in the area between the lungs and between the breastbone and spine
Colonoscopy	An examination of the inside of the colon
Cone biopsy	Remove a cone-shaped piece of tissue from the cervix and cervical canal to diagnosis of cervical cancer
Curettage	Removal of tissue with a curette, a spoon-shaped instrument with a sharp edge
Cystoscopy	Examination of the bladder and urethra using a cystoscope
Dilation and Curettage (D&C)	The cervix is expanded (dilation) and the cervical canal and uterine lining are scraped
Ductal lavage	Collect cells from milk ducts in the breast
Endoscopic retrograde cholangiopancreatography (ERCP)	Endosopic view of gastrointestinal tract to identify abnormalities such as gallstones and pancreatitis
Excisional biopsy	An entire lump or suspicious area is removed for diagnosis
Spinal tap	Lumbar puncture collect cerebrospinal fluid from the lower part of the spinal column using a syringe
Thermal ablation	A procedure using heat to remove tissue or a part of the body, or destroy its function
Thoracoscopy	An endoscope exmination of the inside of the chest used in the diagnosis of lung cancer and other conditions

TABLE 3–6	Treatments That You'll Frequently See in Medical Billing
Treatment	**Description**
Abdominal hysterectomy	Surgical removal of the uterus through the abdomen
Adenoidectomy	Surgical removal of the adenoids
Adjunctive therapy	Secondary treatment given with a primary treatment
Adjuvant therapy	Secondary treatment following a primary treatment
Amputation	Surgery to remove part or all of a limb or appendage
Anastomosis	Connects healthy sections of tubular structures in the body after the diseased portion has been surgically removed
Androgen suppression or androgen ablation	Suppresses or blocks the production of male hormones by surgical removal of the testicles
Anesthesia	Partial or complete loss of sensation, brought on by anasthetic drugs
Angioplasty	Opens clogged arteries
Antibody therapy	Treatment with an antibody to kill tumor cells
Appendectomy	Removals of the appendix
Arthroscopy	A surgical procedure used to diagnose and treat problems inside a joint
Aspiration	Removal of fluid from
Autologous bone marrow transplantation	Bone marrow is removed from a person, stored, and then given back to the person after intensive treatment
Balloon angioplasty	A procedure to open clogged arteries
Biological therapy	Stimulate or restore the ability of the immune system to fight infection and disease
Blepharoplasty	To remove excess fat, along with skin and muscle, from the upper and lower eyelids
Blood transfusion	Administration of blood or blood products into a blood vessel
Bone marrow transplantation	Replaces bone marrow
Brachytherapy	Radiation therapy to treating cancer
Breast-conserving surgery	Removes the breast cancer but not the breast itself

(Continued)

TABLE 3—6 Treatments That You'll Frequently See in Medical Billing (*Continued*)

Treatment	Description
Bypass	Creates a new pathway for the flow of body fluids
C-section	A cesarean section; an incision is made in the uterus to deliver the baby
Cardioversion	Restores the heart beat to a normal rhythm
Carotid endarterectomy	Unclogs the carotid artery
Castration	Removal or destruction of the testicles
Cataract surgery	Removes cataract on eye
Catheterization	A catheter into the body
Cauterization	Destruction of tissue with a hot instrument
Celioscopy	Examines and treats abdominal and pelvic organs using a small surgical viewing instrument called a laparoscope
Cesarean section	An incision is made in a woman's uterus to deliver the baby
Chemoembolization	The blood supply to a tumor is blocked surgically or mechanically and anticancer drugs are administered directly into the tumor
Chemotherapy	Drugs used to treat cancer
Cholecystectomy	Removes the gallbladder
Colectomy	Removes the colon or a portion of the colon
Combination chemotherapy	Treatment using more than one anticancer drug
Complete hysterectomy	The entire uterus, including the cervix
Coronary angioplasty	A balloon is inflated to improve blood flow in the coronary artery
Coronary artery bypass operation	A blood vessel is grafted onto the blocked artery, bypassing the blocked area
Craniotomy	An opening is made in the skull to treat brain tumors
Cryosurgery	Freezing and destroying abnormal tissues
Cryotherapy	Cold temperature to treat disease
Cystectomy	All or part of the bladder treatment of bladder cancer
Decortication	Removal of part or the entire external surface of an organ

(*Continued*)

TABLE 3–6   Treatments That You'll Frequently See in Medical Billing (*Continued*)

Treatment	Description
Dermabrasion	Scraping of the top layers of the skin to reduce wrinkles, acne and other scars
Dialysis	Cleansing the blood when the kidneys are not able to filter the blood
Diathermy	Cauterization, using heat to destroy abnormal cells
Distal pancreatectomy	Removes the body and tail of the pancreas
Endometrial ablation	Removes the lining of the uterus as an alternative to hysterectomy
Endoscopic therapy	Controls bleeding in the treatment of bleeding ulcers, pancreatitis, and other conditions
Epidural block	An anesthetic injected into the space between the wall of the spinal canal and the covering of the spinal cord
Episiotomy	An incision is made between the vagina and the anus to make the vaginal opening larger in order to prevent the area from tearing during labor and delivery
Estrogen replacement therapy (ERT)	Hormones are given to replace the estrogen no longer produced by the ovaries
External-beam radiation	High-energy rays are aimed at the cancer cells
Extracorporeal shock wave lithotripsy	High-energy shockwaves to break up urinary or kidney stones
Fulguration	Using electric current to destroy tissues
Gastrectomy	Removes all or part of the stomach
Gene therapy	Used to alter a gene
General anesthesia	Puts the person to sleep
Hemorrhoidectomy	Removes hemorrhoids
Herniorrhaphy	Repairs a hernia
Horacotomy	Opening the chest used in the diagnosis or treatment of lung cancer and other conditions
Hormonal therapy	Adds, blocks, or removes hormones
Hyperthermic perfusion	Warmed solution containing anticancer drugs passes through the blood vessels of a tumor
Hysterectomy	Removal of the uterus
ICD implantation	Implantation of an implantable cardioverter defibrillator

(*Continued*)

TABLE 3–6   Treatments That You'll Frequently See in Medical Billing (*Continued*)

Treatment	Description
Ileostomy	Opening into the part of the small intestine
Immunosuppression	The body's immune system is suppressed
Implant radiation	Radioactive material placed directly into or near a tumor
Inguinal orchiectomy	Removes testicle through an incision in the groin
Intracarotid infusion	Fluids and drugs administered directly to the carotid artery
Keratectomy	Removal of corneal tissue of the eye
Laminotomy	Removes part of a herniated disk in the spine
Laparoscopic cholecystectomy	Removes the gallbladder
LASIK	Uses a laser to reshape the cornea
LEEP Loop Electrosurgical Excision Procedure	Removal tissue using a hot wire loop
Lithotripsy	Uses high-energy shockwaves to break up gallstones and kidney stones
Lobectomy	Removal of a lobe or portion of an organ
Lumpectomy	Removes the tumor and a small amount of normal tissue around it
Lymphadenectomy	Removes lymph nodes
Mammogram (MAM-o-gram)	X-ray of the breast
Mastectomy	Removes the breast
Metabolic therapy	Corrects changes in metabolism
Microwave therapy	Uses electrodes to generate heat to destroy tissues
Moh's therapy	Treats certain skin cancers
Myectomy	Removes some of the muscles and nerves of the eyelids
Myolysis	Uses electric current or a laser to shrinking of fibroids
Myomectomy	Removes uterine fibroids from the uterus
Nephrectomy	Removes a kidney
Oophorectomy	Removes one or both ovaries
Ovarian ablation	Radiation therapy, or a drug treatment to stop the functioning of the ovaries

(*Continued*)

TABLE 3–6 Treatments That You'll Frequently See in Medical Billing (*Continued*)	
Treatment	**Description**
Pancreaticoduodenectomy	For pancreatic cancer
Patient-controlled analgesia (PCA)	Patient controls when pain medicine is administered
Percutaneous transluminal coronary angioplasty (PTCA)	Opens clogged arteries
Pheresis apheresis	Platelets or white blood cells are taken out of blood and the rest of the blood is returned to the donor
Photodynamic therapy (PDT)	A drug is administered and then activated by light
Photorefractive keratectomy (PRK)	Uses a laser to reshape the stroma of the eye
Pneumonectomy	Removes an entire lung
Prostatectomy	Removes part or all of the prostate
Radial keratotomy	Corrects myopia (nearsightedness)
Radiation surgery	Delivers radiation directly to a tumor while sparing the healthy tissue
Radiation therapy	Uses x-rays, gamma rays, neutrons to kill cancer cells and shrink tumors
Radical cystectomy	Removes the bladder as well as nearby tissues and organs
Radical lymph node dissection	Removes most or all of the lymph nodes that drain lymph from the area around a tumor
Radical mastectomy	Removes which the breast, chest muscles, and all of the lymph nodes under the arm in breast cancer
Radical prostatectomy	Removes the entire prostate
Radiofrequency ablation	Use of electrodes to heat and destroy abnormal tissue
Radiosurgery	Delivers radiation directly to a tumor while sparing the healthy tissue
Radiotherapy	Use of high-energy radiation from x-rays, gamma rays, neutrons to kill cancer cells and shrink tumors
Reconstructive surgery	Reshapes or rebuilds (reconstruct) a part of the body

(Continued)

TABLE 3–6 Treatments That You'll Frequently See in Medical Billing (*Continued*)

Treatment	Description
Refractive surgery	Improves vision by correcting nearsightedness, farsightedness, or astigmatism
Resection	Removal of tissue or of part or all of an organ
Rhinoplasty	Reduces excess cartilage and bone in the nose
Salpinectomy	Removal of one or both fallopian tubes
Salpingo-oophorectomy	Removal of the fallopian tubes and ovaries
Sclerotherapy	Collapsing varicose veins
Spinal Fusion	Two or more vertebrae are fused together
Splenectomy	Removes the spleen
Stem cell transplantation	Replacing immature blood-forming cells that were destroyed by cancer treatment
Stent	A device placed in a body structure to provide support and keep the structure open
Stereotactic radiosurgery	High-dose radiation is administered through openings in the head to a tumor
Steroid therapy	Reduces symptoms of inflammation
Thyroidectomy	Removes part or all of the thyroid
Total Hip Replacement	Replaces the hip joint
Tracheostomy	Creates an opening (stoma) into the windpipe
Transcutaneous electric nerve stimulation (TENS)	Mild electric currents are applied to areas of the skin for pain treatment
Transfusion	The infusion of components of blood or whole blood into the bloodstream
Transplantation	The replacement of an organ with an organ from another person
Transurethral resection (TUR)	Instrument inserted through the urethra to treat enlarged prostate
Urostomy	Making a new way to pass urine following treatment for bladder cancer
Uterine ablation	Removes the lining of the uterus alternative to hysterectomy for treatment of excessive menstrual bleeding
Uterine Fibroid Embolization (UFE)	Cuts off the blood supply to shrink uterine fibroids
Vaginal Hysterectomy	Removal of the uterus through the vagina

Avoid Confusion

Medical words contain clues to their meanings in the form of a prefix, root, and suffix. A prefix is at the beginning of the word. The root is the central part of the word. And the suffix is at the end of the word.

In order to learn the meaning of a word, you must dissect the word into its prefix, root, and suffix. Knowing the meaning of these components of the word enables you to restate them in English words to derive the meaning of the medical word.

You can avoid information overload by learning a few prefixes, roots, and suffixes each day and then trying to find them used in medical articles and advertisements on popular Web sites and publications.

In addition to learning medical words, you'll also need to become familiar with medical tests, procedures, and treatments that are commonly performed by healthcare providers so that you can properly code and bill for them. A *test* is an examination that measures something. A *procedure* is a course of action that achieves a result. And a *treatment* is a type of procedure that relieves illness or injury.

CASE STUDY

CASE 1
The practitioner hands you the results of the patient's examination. It reads: Epigastric pain; dyspepsia; risk for hemorrhage; hypertension. Answer the following questions?

QUESTION 1. What is epigastric pain?
ANSWER: *Gastric* refers to "stomach," *epi* implies "above." Therefore, epigastric pain is pain above the stomach.

QUESTION 2. What is dyspepsia?
ANSWER: *Dys* means bad, difficult, incorrect. *Pepsia* refers to the digestive tract. Dyspepsia means difficult digesting.

QUESTION 3. What is risk for hemorrhage?
ANSWER: *Hem* refers to "blood." *Rrhage* refers to "bursting forward." Risk for hemorrhage refers to the fact that the patient might have in the future blood bursting from a blood vessel.

QUESTION 4. What is hypertension?
ANSWER: *Hyper* means "extreme." *Tension* means "pressure." Hypertension means extreme tension of blood vessels.

FINAL CHECKUP

1. **What is hepatitis?**
   A. Liver inflammation
   B. Hip inflammation
   C. Liver spots on the eyelids
   D. None of the above

2. **Which of the following is inflammation of the gums?**
   A. Gingivitis
   B. Gingivosis
   C. Gingia
   D. Gingivectomy

3. **What is an electroencephalogram?**
   A. Diagram of tissue electrical activity
   B. Recording of tissue electrical activity
   C. Recording of the brain's electrical activity
   D. None of the above

4. **A splenectomy is removal of the spleen.**
   A. True
   B. False

5. **Hemorrhoidectomy is removal of a hernia.**
   A. True
   B. False

6. **A PET scan is a(n)**
   A. Computed image of the metabolic activity of body tissues.
   B. Magnetic resonance imaging (MRI) to measure activity at the cellular level.
   C. X-ray of the hepatic and common bile ducts.
   D. None of the above.

7. **Complete blood count (CBC) is a test used during pregnancy to diagnose birth defects.**
   A. True
   B. False

8. **An angiography is a(n)**

    A. Sample of the amniotic fluid surrounding a fetus.
    B. X-ray scan used to measure the density of your bones.
    C. X-ray of blood vessels.
    D. X-ray of arteries.

9. **Endocarditis in an infection of the outer part of the heart.**

    A. True
    B. False

10. **A colonoscopy is an examination of the inside of the colon.**

    A. True
    B. False

CORRECT ANSWERS AND RATIONALES

1. A. Liver inflammation.
2. A. Gingivitis.
3. C. Recording of the brain's electrical activity.
4. A. True.
5. B. False.
6. A. Computed image of the metabolic activity of body tissues.
7. B. False.
8. C. X-ray of blood vessels.
9. B. False.
10. A. True.

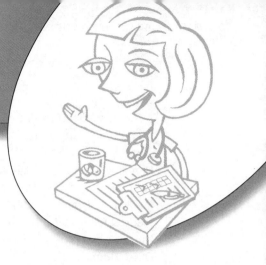

chapter 4

Medical Office Procedures

KEY TERMS

A Group Medical Practice
Ambulatory Care Center
Clinic
Handling Emergency Calls
Hospital
Medical Assistant
Medical Technicians
Nurses
Office Hours

Physician Assistants and Nurse
  Practitioners
Practitioners
Registered Health Information
  Technician
Retail Clinic
Single-Practitioner Medical Practice
Transferring a Call
Urgent Care Clinic

1. Behind the Scenes

There's not much to do while sitting in the waiting room except to watch your doctor and his healthcare team go about their business—all the time scratching your head wondering what they are doing.

As a medical insurance specialist, you'll be part of that healthcare team. In this chapter, you'll learn about the responsibilities of each team member and how the team members interact with each other. You'll also learn procedures that are commonly used in every medical practice.

Working for a medical practice can be confusing at first especially for anyone who has worked for a hospital or for a large organization in private industry because a medical practice uses procedures that are different from other businesses.

A medical practice is a relatively small business that is owned and operated by one or more practitioners. A practitioner opens a medical practice after completing 4 years of medical school and 3 years of closely supervised training in a hospital, known as a *residency*. By this time in their career, practitioners have the medical skills a medical practice demands, but may lack the business know-how to run a successful practice.

After completing their residency, some practitioners join an existing medical practice as an employee before opening their own medical practice. Others partner with fellow practitioners to open a group medical practice. Still others choose to work for healthcare facilities such as hospitals; ambulatory centers referred to as urgent care centers; or clinics.

Single-Practitioner Medical Practice

A **single-practitioner medical practice** is owned and operated by a practitioner who is responsible for the healthcare of his/her patients and for running the medical practice as a profitable business. The practitioner might provide family care; focus on a specialty such as geriatrics; or provide a combination of family care and a specialty.

The major advantage of working for a single-practitioner medical practice is the opportunity to take on different roles on the healthcare team. Since there is one practitioner, the number of patients cared for by the medical practice is relatively small compared with that of a group medical practice. It is for this reason that this type of medical practice supports only a few employees. Each one has to take on more than one responsibility.

The major disadvantage of working for a single-practitioner medical practice is the lack of structure that is found in a group practice or larger healthcare organization. Aside from legal requirements, the structure of a single-practitioner medical practice is totally at the practitioner's discretion. Titles, job descriptions, salaries, raises, promotions, vacations, sick leaves, work schedules, and benefits can differ from practice to practice—and can change at any time without warning.

A Group Medical Practice

A **group medical practice** is owned and operated by two or more practitioners who are responsible for patient care. They delegate the business aspects of the practice to an office manager whose job is to create a structure for the medical practice to run efficiently and profitably. One practitioner is designated as the manager of the practice who with the advice and consent of the other practitioners hires the staff and is involved in important administrative decisions such as office leases, salaries, and computer systems. Under this practitioner is the office manager who handles the day-to-day operations.

The major advantage of working for a group medical practice is its structure and stability and ability to focus on one area of the medical practice. The patient load provides the workload and income to hire a full staff including a medical insurance specialist. Titles, job descriptions, salaries, raises, promotions, vacations, sick leaves, work schedules, and benefits are provided based on those offered by similar size group practices. Group practices try to maintain a competitive structure in order to retain a good staff.

The major disadvantage of working for a group medical practice is the inflexibility for support, training, and career advancement. Staff members are expected to perform their job accurately and independently with little or no support. For example, there might be one medical insurance specialist on staff who is responsible for processing all the claims for the group medical practice without any assistance. Furthermore, the group medical practice is too small to offer training and career development for the staff. Since there are few duplicate roles in the organization, there are limited opportunities for anyone to transfer to a different job.

Ambulatory Care Center

An **ambulatory care center** is usually owned and operated by a corporation, such as a medical insurer or healthcare maintenance organization, and might be part of a chain of centers in a state, metropolitan region, or across the nation. An ambulatory care center operates similar to an emergency room, a clinic, or other department of a hospital. Practitioners are their full-time or per diem employees and probably don't have a financial interest in the center.

The major advantage of working for an ambulatory care center is the greater structure and stability than is found in a group practice plus there is the opportunity for career development and job transfer especially in centers that are part of a chain. The structure and stability are similar to a hospital. The opportunity for career development and job transfer exceeds that of a hospital in some cases because a chain has multiple healthcare facilities that are joined together by a single infrastructure (ie, computer systems, centralized management, departments that service multiple centers).

The major disadvantage of working for an ambulatory care center is its inflexibility. Operating decisions and procedures are typically set for the entire chain of centers by off-site managers who are focused on the bottom line. The office manager of a particular center has less discretion than the office manager of a group practice.

Clinic

A *clinic* is a specialized practice that can be owned and operated by a group of practitioners or by a large healthcare organization such as a hospital. Practitioners who work at a clinic have the same medical interests. Examples of clinics are baby wellness centers, sports injury clinics, women's health clinics, and rehabilitation facilities.

The major advantage of working for a clinic is that you become highly proficient in a specialty, which reduces the opportunity for errors. For example, a medical insurance specialist has the opportunity to become an expert in processing sports injury claims if he works for a sports injury clinic.

The major disadvantage of working for a clinic is its self-limiting opportunities for career growth because you are exposed to only that area of specialty. That is, you might be an expert in claims for sports injuries, but your skills for processing other claims are lost.

Urgent Care Clinic

Urgent care clinic is a walk-in clinic that delivers ambulatory care and provides an alternative to relatively minor care handled by traditional emergency room. Urgent care centers treat injuries and illnesses that require immediate care but not emergency care.

Urgent care centers are typically owned by a group of practitioners; however, there is a trend for corporations and investment banks acquiring urgent care centers in an effort to create brands that are marketed to consumers.

Some consumers believe that urgent care centers provide a lower quality care because they are staffed mainly by non-physician practitioner providers and a high turnover rate of staff. The RAND corporation reported that consumers rate the quality at retail clinics highest, followed by urgent care clinics, then doctor's offices and emergency rooms.

Retail Clinic

A **retail (or convenient) care clinic** can be found in retail stores such as pharmacies and large super stores. A retail care clinic provides care for minor illnesses and minor preventive care such as flu shots. Non-physician practitioner providers, such as medical assistants, nurses, and nurse practitioners (NPs), provide care.

Hospital

A *hospital* is a large healthcare facility that offers outpatient and inpatient care. Most hospitals offer the same breadth of services, while some also offer specialty care such as cardiac surgery, burns, and major trauma care. Hospitals are owned by a public or private corporation and employ practitioners on a salary or per diem basis.

The major advantage of working for a hospital is that it has a highly structured work environment that offers an opportunity to grow into positions. For example, many hospitals offer entry-level positions for medical insurance specialists giving them the opportunity to gain experience under the direction of a more senior medical insurance specialist.

The major disadvantage of working for a hospital is the lack of opportunity to interact with patients. In a single-practitioner private practice and a group practice, and to an extent with ambulatory centers and clinics, a medical insurance specialist discusses insurance coverage with patients. This associates a real person with the claim. However, in a hospital setting it is easy to lose this connection, resulting in the claim becoming just another piece of paper.

2. The Healthcare Team

As a medical insurance specialist you'll be working with other members of the healthcare team to provide care for patients. Although a medical insurance specialist doesn't care directly for patients, he/she is still an important player on the healthcare team because reimbursements for medical claims he/she processes provide the financial resources to care for patients.

The healthcare team consists of practitioners, practitioner assistants, NPs, nurses, medical technicians, medical records specialists, medical assistants, and medical insurance specialists.

Practitioners

A *practitioner* is a medical professional whose responsibility is to examine patients and diagnose and treat illnesses. Practitioners can be placed into two categories: general practitioner or specialist. A general practitioner is a primary care practitioner who handles examinations and routine illnesses. A specialist is a practitioner who focuses on a related group of illnesses.

For example, a patient visits his primary care practitioner if he has a persistent cough. The primary care practitioner examines the patient and may take a chest X-ray. If unexpected spots appear on the X-ray, the patient is referred to a practitioner who specializes in respiratory illnesses where the patient undergoes an additional examination and tests to narrow the diagnosis and treatment.

Physician Assistants and Nurse Practitioners

Physician assistants (PAs) and NPs are medical professionals who are licensed to perform some of a practitioner's duties under the direct supervision of a practitioner. Each state sets the licensing requirements for PAs and NPs; however, typically they have a 4-year degree and advanced medical training.

Their duties are established by state law and by the practitioner who oversees their work. However, most are permitted to perform physical examinations, order medical tests, write prescriptions, and diagnose and treat many routine illnesses.

PAs and NPs are referred to as *practitioner extenders* because they are able to provide patients with routine healthcare while the practitioner cares for more serious cases.

Typically, the PA or NP will be the first member of the healthcare team to assess the condition of a new patient or an existing patient who is presenting with a new illness. They work up the patient and then arrive at a preliminary diagnosis and treatment, which they present to the practitioner.

For minor illnesses such as a head cold or an upper respiratory infection, the practitioner may briefly visit the patient to confirm the findings before signing off on the diagnosis and treatment. Sometimes the practitioner might simply approve treatment without seeing the patient if the condition is routine. However, the PA and NP immediately turn the patient over to the practitioner at the first signs of a more serious illness.

Nurses

Nurses are members of the healthcare team who are licensed to observe, assess, and record a patient's symptoms. They can dispense medication, perform certain medical procedures, and provide medical advice to patients and their families once the practitioner, PA, or NP reaches a medical diagnosis and prescribes medication or treatment.

There are generally three types of licensed nurses: **registered nurse** (RN), **licensed practical nurse** (LPN), and NP that was discussed in the previous section. Requirements for a license are established by each state. Typically, an RN must complete at least a 2-year training program and an LPN a 1-year training program. Both have to pass state licensing examinations commonly referred to as *the boards*. Many RNs also have 2- or 4-year nursing degrees.

Medical Technicians

Medical technicians perform advanced diagnostic and treatment procedures and laboratory tests ordered by the practitioner, PA, or NP. These professionals fall into one of many categories, each having its own medical title.

For example, a phlebotomist is a medical technician who draws blood from patients to be used in blood tests performed by medical laboratory technicians. Likewise, an X-ray technician is a medical technician who takes X-rays of patients.

Medical technicians undergo different types of training depending on their specialty. For example, a phlebotomist and ECG technician may go through several months of training, while it takes 2 years to complete an X-ray technician program. A laboratory technician must complete 2 to 4 years of training.

Registered Health Information Technician

Observations, medical or surgical interventions, and treatment outcomes are recorded each time a patient receives healthcare. It is the registered health information technician's responsibility to ensure that the patient's medical records are complete and accurate. The registered health information technician must make sure that the patient's medical chart, medical forms, and computerized records are updated immediately. The practitioner and other members of the healthcare team who treated the patient are asked to clarify any information that isn't clear to the registered health information technician.

An important responsibility for the registered health information technician may be to properly code the patient's treatment in order for the practitioner and the healthcare team to be reimbursed by the patient's medical insurer. Each diagnosis and procedure performed on the patient must be coded based on the patient's medical records and diagnosis and procedure classification manuals.

Registered health information technicians are assisted by other healthcare professionals who code insurance claims. These professionals are called health information coders, medical record coders, coders/abstractors, or coding specialists.

Medical records specialist's training requires a 2-year degree (AA) in Health Information Management. Then the registered health information technician is qualified to take the certification test given by the American Health Information Management Association.

Medical Assistant

A *medical assistant* is a member of the healthcare team who has a variety of responsibilities in the medical office including acting as a receptionist, appointment scheduler as well as a medical billing specialist. A medical assistant may also focus on one function within the medical office such as medical transcriptions. Practitioners usually record their notes about a patient. The medical assistant then transcribes those notes using a word processor, and the notes are then entered into the patient's record.

Some medical assistants are given the responsibility to welcome the patient, collect general information and insurance information from the patient, gather the patient's medical records, and escort the patient to the examination room. They are also responsible for scheduling treatment, scheduling a new appointment, taking care of payment, and updating the patient's records before the patient leaves the office.

Training for a medical assistant varies from on-the-job training to a year of formal training and certification by the American Association of Medical Assistants or National Health Career Association.

3. Medical Office Procedures

You have visited a medical office and therefore probably have some idea of the office procedures—at least from the patient's point of view. Now let's take a behind-the-scenes look at what goes on before, during, and after a patient's visit.

Each practitioner has his own policy for seeing and treating patients. Medical assistants and other members of the healthcare team are expected to learn and enforce this policy. This can be challenging in a group practice because the policy may differ for each practitioner in the group.

This policy is the basis for establishing office hours. Office hours are the times that the practitioner is available to see patients in the office. Practitioners juggle office hours around other activities such as hospital rounds and time off.

Office Hours

Medical office hours vary based on the type of medical practice and patient needs. For example, a large family medical practice could be open 12 hours a day, 6 days a week; an urgent care center is open 24 hours a day, 7 days a week; and a surgical practice might be open 5 hours a day for pre- and postoperative consultations.

Office hours are scheduled to reduce waiting times for patients and to make the best use of the healthcare team's time. There are six types of office hours.

1. **Fixed office hours**. Some medical practices set fixed office hours during which a practitioner—or other members of the healthcare team—is available to see patients. No appointment is necessary. This avoids the difficulties that are common when scheduling appointments such as patients not showing for their appointment. A major disadvantage of fixed office hours is wasted time. Few or no patients might visit. Another disadvantage is that the practitioner is unable to anticipate the time spent with each patient because he/she doesn't know what their condition is until he/she sees them in the examination room. As a result patients may have long waiting times to see the practitioner.

2. **Scheduled appointments**. Other medical practices require scheduled appointments. A practitioner provides the medical assistant a block of time when he/she is available. The assistant then arranges appointments with patients. The nature of a patient's request determines the length of an appointment. This enables the medical assistant to reduce patients' waiting times. Although scheduling appointments makes the best use of the practitioner's time, it does have two important disadvantages. First, a patient may not keep the appointment. This can impact revenue for the medical practice since the patient is charged only for visits—not for missed appointments. The other disadvantage is the increased length of time it takes for a patient to see a practitioner. A patient who is sick today doesn't want to wait for 2 weeks for an appointment and therefore will look for another primary care practitioner.

3. **Wave scheduling**. Wave scheduling blends the best of fixed office hours and scheduling appointments. In wave scheduling the practitioner provides the medical assistant with a block of time when he/she is available to see patients. However, only a portion of this time is allocated to scheduled patients. The other time slots are allotted to walk-in patients. Here's how this works. Let's say six patients are scheduled per hour averaging 10 minutes per patient. The practitioner probably sees each patient for less than 10 minutes because the first few minutes are spent with the nurse who assesses the patient prior to the practitioner's examination and diagnosis. The practitioner then turns the patient back over to the nurse and medical technician for treatment and required medical tests while he/she moves on to the next patient. The practitioner may revisit the patient after reviewing the medical tests.

4. **Double booking**. The double-booking scheduling method gives two and sometimes three patients the same appointment with a practitioner. It is assumed that all three patients won't arrive at the same time thereby creating a natural buffer between patients. The major disadvantage is that patients will have to wait to see the practitioner even though they arrive on time for their appointment.

5. **Computer scheduling**. Computer software schedules appointments for the medical assistant based on the nature of the patient's complaint and the block of time available in the practitioner's schedule. Besides scheduling appointments, the software also sends a confirmation notice via e-mail to the patient, prints a daily schedule for the practitioner, and generates various reports such as those indicating which patients failed to keep their appointment without notifying the office.

6. **Out-of-office appointments**. The medical assistant also schedules out-of-office appointments for patients such as for diagnostic tests and treatments that can only be performed in a hospital. Likewise, when a practitioner refers a patient to a specialist, the medical assistant typically schedules these visits for the patient.

4. Telephone Calls

A medical practice receives a variety of calls from patients, pharmacies, hospitals, medical laboratories, healthcare providers, medical insurers, government agencies, and sales representatives each having a different request. Everyone associated with the medical practice is trained to respond to these requests.

Incoming phone calls should be promptly answered, usually on the second ring. The caller is greeted by saying slowly the proper name of the practice such as "Main Street Medical Practice" or "Dr. Robert Smith's office." Slang names, such as Main Street Medical or Dr. Bob's office, are not used. Likewise it is improper to simply say "doctor's office" because the doctor isn't identified, which can lead to confusion. The patient may make the appointment not realizing he/she called the wrong practitioner.

Following the greeting the caller is asked, "How can I help you" or "How may I direct your call?" Some medical practices require the caller to be asked, "Is this an emergency?" If so, the call is then immediately transferred to a nurse or other licensed healthcare provider.

If it isn't an emergency, then the call is screened. The objective of screening a call is to determine the appropriate action to take based on the practitioner's policy. Here's how to screen a call. Ask the caller what the nature of the call is. This gives a clue as to who can help the caller. And then ask the caller for key information about the nature of his call. Key information is information needed to understand the caller's request. If the caller is

- A **patient scheduling an appointment**. Ask for the patient's name, address, and telephone number and whether or not she is a new patient.
- A **pharmacy calling about a prescription**. Ask for the pharmacist's name, pharmacy name, telephone number, patient's name, and pharmacist's question.
- A **medical testing service calling about a patient**. Ask for the caller's name, company name, telephone number, patient's name, and the nature of the test.
- A **healthcare provider**. Ask for the person's name and who the person is calling for.
- A **sales representative**. Ask for the person's name, the company name, telephone number, and the product he is selling.
- An **insurer**. Ask for the person's name, company name, telephone number, and claims number.

Transferring a Call

The person who answers the call is responsible for either personally handling the caller's request or transferring the caller to the proper person. The policy of the practice will determine who handles a request.

When transferring a call, tell the caller the name of the person to whom you are transferring the call. Place the call on hold, and then call your colleague and tell him/her who is calling and the nature of the call. Also provide your colleague with key information that you gathered from the caller. This helps him/her prepare for the call.

If possible, stay on the line until the call is transferred and then introduce the caller to your colleague by saying, "I have Mrs. Smith on the phone for you." Hang up as soon as their conversation begins.

Projecting a Telephone Image

Your voice projects an image of you and the medical practice in the caller's mind. A good speaking voice and the proper telephone etiquette convey that you are a professional and capable of addressing the caller's needs.

Here are some tips to consider when handling callers:

- Speak in clear, pleasant tones to convey self-assurance.
- Show a sincere interest in the caller's request.
- Focus only on the caller and avoid doing other things while on the phone.
- Listen carefully.
- Ask the caller to clarify anything that you don't understand.
- Each call is an opportunity to present a positive image of the medical practice to the caller.
- Take accurate notes including key information. Make sure to use correct spelling. Ask the caller to spell words that you don't know how to spell.
- Take ownership of the request and stay with the caller until you find the right colleague to help him/her.
- Be patient regardless of how busy it is in the office.
- Give the caller time to understand what you are saying.
- Avoid medical jargon. Instead use terms that are easily understood by the caller.
- Keep the call short and to the point without giving the caller the feeling that he/she is being rushed off the phone.
- Speak properly and don't use slang.

Handling Emergency Calls

As strange as it may seem, some patients call their family practitioner rather than dialing 911 in a healthcare emergency, and as a result everyone in the medical practice must know how to respond to an emergency call.

The caller will likely be upset and may find it difficult to focus on the phone call. When the caller seems disoriented, assume that it is an emergency call. Your job is to stay calm and give the caller specific directions.

Here's what to do:

- Ask, "What is the nature of the emergency?"
- Ask, "What is the address of the emergency?"
- Ask, "What is the caller's telephone number?"
- Tell the caller to remain on the line. Don't put the caller on hold.

- Use another telephone line to call 911. Identify yourself to the 911 operator and explain the situation. Give the 911 operator the address of the emergency and the caller's telephone. Follow the directions of the 911 operator.

- Ask a colleague to have a licensed healthcare provider (practitioner, nurse, practitioner assistant, NP) join the call.

Preparing to Return a Call

Except for patient appointments and administrative inquiries, many calls must be returned because they come in when the practitioner is with patients. Each call is important, and an effort should be made to return the call on the same day or at the beginning of the next day.

When a caller's request cannot be addressed immediately, detailed information about the request is written as part of a message given to the person who will respond to the call. The message should contain sufficient information so the person can respond with an answer.

Let's say a pharmacist calls asking if he/she can substitute a generic drug for the brand name drug prescribed by the practitioner. Besides noting the key information described previously in this chapter, you'll also need to make note of the name and manufacturer of the generic drug and maybe the price difference between the generic and the brand name. This and key information is placed in the message to the practitioner. The practitioner can review the technical information about the generic drug before returning the call.

Be sure to place the date and time on the message and make note of the message in a notebook. The notebook is a record of the call and is used as a reminder and a backup in case the original message is misplaced.

Give the caller an estimate of when to expect the return call. Some practitioners set aside periods during the day to return calls, while others prioritize calls and respond to the most urgent calls between patient visits.

Here are tips for taking messages:

- Write neatly.

- Ask the caller to spell words that you don't know how to spell.

- Don't paraphrase the call. The message should be in the caller's words to avoid miscommunication.

- Don't respond yourself unless you are authorized to respond.

- Don't acknowledge a patient or release any patient information over the phone. Simply say that you'll pass along the message to the appropriate person.

- Read the complete message back to the caller including the spelling of any word you don't know how to spell.
- Ask the caller if he/she is under a time constraint. For example, the patient may be waiting while the pharmacist is on the phone.
- Tell the person who is returning the call about any time constraints.
- Don't promise something you can't deliver. Don't say the practitioner will return the call in a half hour unless the practitioner tells you to do so.
- Keep the message brief and to the point.

Follow the policy of the medical practice for delivering the message. Some practices require that the message be written on a form and then organized into piles such as patient, laboratories, pharmacies, sales representative, personal, or other. The practitioner can then scan through these piles and return the most urgent calls.

Other practices require that the patient's chart be pulled and attached to the message before being reviewed by the practitioner. In this way the practitioner has all the information at hand to respond to the caller.

Many times a copy of the message is placed in the patient's chart along with the practitioner's response. The practitioner—and anyone authorized to view the patient's medical records—can piece together what transpired during the phone call.

5. The Answering Service

Patients may call a medical practice anytime day or night, weekends, or holidays. The office staff doesn't work during all these hours. Instead an answering service, available 24 hours a day, 7 days a week, answers the telephone calls whenever the office is closed.

Service personnel at the answering service are trained to screen calls and take messages. Messages taken by the answering service are less detailed than messages taken by the office staff. The answering service simply notes the date and time of the call, who called, and the caller's telephone number. Depending on the practitioner, the answering service may contact the practitioner by phone or pager or may wait for the practitioner to call the answering service for messages.

Answering services might also respond to simple questions from the caller such as inquiries about office hours.

6. Making Calls on Behalf of the Medical Practice

Medical assistants and others on the staff are frequently required to make calls to patients, hospitals, insurers, laboratories, and others who work directly or indirectly with the practice. Each call should be planned before the call is made to avoid wasting time. Establish an outcome for the call. Gather pertinent information that might be needed during the call. Know the name or department of the person you are calling.

Let's say you have been asked to arrange a hospital admission for a patient. The outcome of the call is confirmation that the hospital is prepared to admit the patient. Before making the call you need to gather the patient's complete name, age, date of birth, address, telephone number, diagnosis, previous admissions to the hospital, preferred date for admission to the hospital, and special accommodations that the patient requires.

If the patient is going for surgery or a diagnostic procedure, you'll also need to know the type of surgery and other procedures to be performed on the patient, length of time needed for the surgery, surgical assistance required, type of anesthesia, and any other special requirements.

Be prepared to document the call. Note the date and time you called and the name, title, and phone number of each person you called along with questions you asked and their responses. Verify their response by reading back your notes. Some medical practices require that notes of calls pertaining to a patient be placed in the patient's medical record, while other medical practices leave it to the discretion of the staff member as to how the notes are stored.

For example, the hospital admitting staff will give you instructions for the patient, which contain the date and time that the patient is to arrive and who to meet in the admitting office. There might be additional instructions depending on the nature of the patient's hospital visit. For example, the patient might be required to visit the laboratory for preadmission testing before the admitting date. Likewise the patient may be told not to eat or drink anything 24 hours before being admitted.

7. Medical Records

A *medical record* is a permanent document that contains the medical history of a patient. It contains general information such as the patient's name, address, phone number, employer, and insurer. It also contains the results of previous visits, examinations, prescriptions, laboratory tests, and treatments. An entry in a patient's medical record is the basis for future diagnosis and treatment and reimbursement from a medical insurer.

Medical records are stored in a file system that gives the office staff quick access to any patient's medical record within a few minutes. Before a medical record is stored, it is inspected for accuracy and completeness. Each document within the medical record is reviewed to ensure it is in good physical condition.

The inspection also determines whether there are outstanding issues that must still be addressed. For example, the practitioner's notes may still need to be transcribed or a laboratory result may not have been received as yet. Depending on the policy of the medical practice, a medical record might not be returned to the file until those outstanding issues are resolved.

Once the inspection is completed, the medical record is released. The release process differs with each practice but usually entails that a note be included on the medical record indicating the date and time and with the initials of the person who inspected it.

The medical record is then stored using its primary key. A primary key is information contained in a patient's medical record that is used to retrieve it. For example, a patient's name could be a primary key.

Some medical filing systems have a way of cross-referencing medical records. A cross-reference is an alternative way to identify a medical record. For example, each patient's record is assigned a patient identity (ID) number that can be used in place of the patient's name to protect the patient's confidentiality. A medical filing system may cross-reference patient IDs with patient names. A medical assistant can look up a patient's name in the cross-reference to locate the patient's ID if it isn't available.

Patient information is stored in reverse chronological order in the patient's medical record. The most current information is at the beginning of the medical record.

Types of Medical Filing Systems

There are many types of filing systems available to manage medical records. These include alphabetical, numeric, subject.

- **Alphabetical**. This is the most popular system used for storing medical information because it organizes medical records by the patient's last name and first name making it easy to locate a patient's medical record when he/she arrives for the appointment. The lack of confidentiality is the major disadvantage for using this system because the patient's name is in clear sight.

- **Numeric**. A numeric filing system requires that each patient be assigned a unique number which is used as the primary way of finding a patient's medical record. This addresses the confidentiality problem exhibited in the alphabetical system because only the patient's ID number is visible on the outside of the medical record. The disadvantage of a numeric filing system is that the patient's ID can be inadvertently transposed. Patient IDs are assigned using the straight-numeric method or the terminal digit method. The straight-numeric method assigns patients a number in sequential order with the first number assigned to the first patient. The terminal digit method divides numbers into sections. Sections define a group of patients. Here is an example of a terminal digit number that is divided into three sections: 2008-01-35. The first section is 2008 and represents the year. The second section is 01 and represents a practitioner within the group practice. And 35 represents the patient. The patient's ID number is 2008-01-35 indicating that he/she is the 35th patient of practitioner 01 who started coming to the practice in 2008.

- **Subject**. A subject filing system organizes patient information according to subject area such as patient information, insurer, and medical records and provides a more efficient way to maintain information and ensure confidentiality. For example, the status of a patient's account is contained under the patient information subject. Likewise, outstanding claims from a particular insurer are found under the insurer category. The advantage of this method is that everything related to one subject is in one location. The disadvantage is deciding where to file information. Some information could fit into more than one subject area—or none of the existing subject areas—and as a result the information might be difficult to locate quickly. Cross-referencing is frequently used to address this concern.

- **Color coding**. A color-coding filing system uses colored folders to organize patient records or colored labels can be used to represent the patient's name or ID number. Color coding is a device used in conjunction with the above filing systems to make retrieval of the medical record easier. Each color represents a series of letters of the alphabet such as red for letters A through D; yellow for letters E through H, and so on.

Tips on Filing

Maintaining medical records is critical to the success of a medical practice and to the healthcare of patients. Misplacing a medical record could be life-threatening because information it contains is used to determine the proper treatment for the patient. Let's say an elderly person is being treated for an infection. The practitioner might prescribe penicillin, if the patient isn't allergic to penicillin. The patient's medical records contain his allergies. The patient is at risk if his medical records are not available to the practitioner.

Here are some ways to reduce the likelihood of misfiling patient records.

- Alphabetize all letters and not simply the first few letters.
- Ignore punctuation marks when alphabetizing.
- Don't file anything that isn't properly labeled.
- Numbers come before alphabetical characters.
- File according to last name, first name, and middle name.
- Names of businesses, institutions, and organizations are filed according to the way the name is written. File "Bob Smith & Company" as "Bob Smith & Company" and not "Smith, Bob, & Company."
- File using symbols and coordinating words in a name such as *the*, *a*, and #. File "The Bob Smith & Company" as "Bob Smith & Company" and not "The Bob Smith & Company."
- Ignore apostrophes. File "Bob's" as "Bobs."
- Place titles last. File "Dr. Smith" as "Smith, Dr."
- File hyphenated names as one unit such as in the case of married women who choose to use both their maiden and married name. Mary Smith-Jones should be filed as "SmithJones, Mary."
- Combine prefixes and roots. File "Bob Van der Hooke" as "Vanderhooke, Bob."
- Use the city and state to file if two names are the same.
- Seniority designations such as Sr. and Jr. should be filed in alphabetic order. File "Bob Smith Jr." and then "Bob Smith Sr."
- Names that contain numbers are placed in numerical order. File, "10th Avenue Deli" first followed by "12th Avenue Deli."
- Don't use abbreviations. File "U.S. Treasury Department" as "United States Treasury Department."

CASE STUDY

CASE 1

The medical billing specialist applied for a position in a group practice setting and is called for an interview. The medical billing specialist is interviewed by the office manager and each of the five principal practitioners of the group. They ask the following questions. What is the best response?

QUESTION 1. What is wave scheduling?

ANSWER: In wave scheduling the practitioner provides the medical assistant with a block of time when he/she is available to see patients. However, only a portion of this time is allocated to scheduled patients. The other time slots are allotted to walk-in patients. Here's how this works. Let's say six patients are scheduled per hour averaging 10 minutes per patient. The practitioner probably sees each patient for less than 10 minutes because the first few minutes are spent with the nurse who assesses the patient prior to the practitioner's examination and diagnosis. The practitioner then turns the patient back over to the nurse and medical technician for treatment and required medical tests while he/she moves on to the next patient. The practitioner may revisit the patient after reviewing the medical tests.

QUESTION 2. Why do practices use double-booking scheduling patients?

ANSWER: The double-booking scheduling method gives two and sometimes three patients the same appointment with a practitioner. It is assumed that all three patients won't arrive at the same time thereby creating a natural buffer between patients. The major disadvantage is that patients will have to wait to see the practitioner even though they arrive on time for their appointment.

QUESTION 3. How would you handle an emergency telephone call from a patient?

ANSWER: Do the following:

Ask, "What is the nature of the emergency?"

Ask, "What is the address of the emergency?"

Ask, "What is the caller's telephone number?"

Tell the caller to remain on the line. Don't put the caller on hold.

Use another telephone line to call 911. Identify yourself to the 911 operator and explain the situation. Give the 911 operator the address of the emergency and the caller's telephone. Follow the directions of the 911 operator.

Ask a colleague to have a licensed healthcare provider (practitioner, nurse, practitioner assistant, nurse practitioner) join the call.

QUESTION 4. What is a color-coding filing system?

ANSWER: A color-coding filing system uses colored folders to organize patient records or colored labels can be used to represent the patient's name or ID number. Color coding is a device used in conjunction with other filing systems to make retrieval of the medical record easier. Each color represents a series of letters of the alphabet such as red for letters A through D; yellow for letters E through H, and so on.

FINAL CHECKUP

1. **When you determine a call is an emergency, ask**
   A. What is the nature of the emergency?
   B. What is the address of the emergency?
   C. What is the caller's telephone number?
   D. All of the above.

2. **The scheduling method that gives the same appointment to two or more patients is called**
   A. Computer scheduling
   B. Double booking
   C. Wave scheduling
   D. None of the above

3. **A practitioner's assistant is**
   A. Licensed to perform some of a practitioner's duties under the direct supervision of a practitioner.
   B. A phlebotomist.
   C. Responsible in the medical office.
   D. All of the above.

4. **Office hours are scheduled to reduce waiting times for patients and make the best use of the healthcare team's time.**
   A. True
   B. False

5. **When a caller's request cannot be addressed immediately, detailed information about the request is written as part of a message given to the person who will respond to the call.**
   A. True
   B. False

6. **Patient information is filed using the**

    A. Alphabetical filing system

    B. Numeric filing system

    C. Color-coding filing system

    D. All of the above

7. **Nurses are members of the healthcare team who are licensed to observe, assess, and record a patient's symptoms.**

    A. True

    B. False

8. **The member of the healthcare team who is responsible for maintaining, storing, and retrieving patient records is the**

    A. Phlebotomist

    B. Medical technician

    C. Medical records specialist

    D. None of the above

9. **With fixed office hours, patients do not require an appointment to see the practitioner.**

    A. True

    B. False

10. **Speak in clear, pleasant tones to convey self-assurance when answering the telephone.**

    A. True

    B. False

CORRECT ANSWERS AND RATIONALES

1. D. All of the above.
2. B. Double booking.
3. A. Licensed to perform some of a practitioner's duties under the direct supervision of a practitioner .
4. A. True.
5. A. True.
6. D. All of the above.
7. A. True.
8. C. Medical records specialist.
9. B. False.
10. A. True.

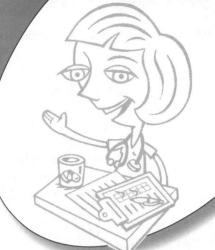

chapter **5**

Introduction to Procedural Coding

1. Here's How Coding Works

It's time to roll up your sleeves, sit down, and dig into learning how billing codes are used to pay for medical procedures, such as checkups by your doctor, and medical services such as the ambulance ride to your hospital.

There are countless medical procedures and services that healthcare professionals provide to patients every day and each is charged separately. What an administrative nightmare—that is, if it wasn't for a coding system that streamlines claims processing so that computers can handle most claims with little human intervention.

However, computers can process claims only if the medical insurance specialist enters the proper billing code on the claim. And as you'll soon learn, finding the correct code requires special knowledge of the billing code system, medicine, and rules set by medical insurers.

A patient visits her physician complaining about pain in the midchest area after she ate a big meal. The physician must diagnose and treat if possible. First, he rules out heart problems by conducting an electrocardiogram (ECG). If the results are negative for any anomalies, the doctor may request an X-ray to take a look inside the patient.

The X-ray shows a small unusual mass in the area slightly below the liver. The physician needs to take a piece of the mass, called a *specimen,* to test it, so he orders a biopsy. The patient is anesthetized and a needle is inserted to remove a small piece of the mass, which is sent to the pathology laboratory for study.

The pathology laboratory reports that the mass is benign. The physician then refers the patient to a surgeon. The surgeon examines the patient and reviews the X-ray and laboratory results and then schedules the patient for outpatient surgery in the hospital. The surgeon performs a laparoscopic procedure to remove the mass. Three small incisions are made, the mass is removed, and the patient goes home the same day.

Up to a week or so before surgery, the patient undergoes a series of blood tests—standard for any patient scheduled for surgery. The patient reports to the hospital early in the morning on the day of the surgery. She is prepped and wheeled into the operating room. After the surgery, she returns to her room where she is cared for until she recovers enough to go home.

The patient has scheduled follow-up visits with the surgeon and then with her physicians for the week after the surgery. They examine her, and if all is well, she is formally discharged, which means that she is healed.

2. Getting Paid

Her physician, the pathology laboratory, her surgeon, and the hospital need to get paid for her care. Typically, the patient's health insurer pays healthcare providers directly. In order to be paid, healthcare providers must submit a claim form to the health insurer. This is the job of the medical insurance specialist.

This case results in five claims. These are submitted by the physician, the pathology laboratory, the surgeon, the anesthesiologist, and the hospital. Each claim is prepared by a medical insurance specialist and must state the date the care was given, the code that represents the procedure or service rendered, and the rate, which is the price charged by the healthcare provider.

As you can imagine there are thousands of different procedures and services that healthcare providers can perform when caring for a patient. Here is a list of the procedures and services used to care for the patient in our example.

- The initial office visit with the physician.
- The ECG.
- The X-ray.
- Anesthesia for the biopsy.
- The biopsy.
- The pathology and laboratory examination of the specimen.
- The second office visit to discuss the results of the laboratory findings.
- The initial office visit with the surgeon.
- The surgeon's examination of the X-ray and laboratory reports.

- Laboratory tests before the surgery.
- The surgery.
- Follow-up office visits with the physician and the surgeon.

Each procedure and service is identified by a unique code, which makes it easy for healthcare providers to submit claims and for insurers to process claims. These codes are defined in the **Healthcare Common Procedure Coding System** (HCPCS).

3. The Healthcare Common Procedure Coding System

The HCPCS is the standardized coding system used to process Medicare and health insurance claims for payment. It consists of two subsystems referred to as *Level I* and *Level II*.

Level I is referred to as the *Current Procedural Terminology* (CPT) and associates the descriptions of procedures and services performed by physicians and other healthcare providers with a unique five-digit numeric code. CPT is maintained by the American Medical Association (AMA).

Level II, referred to as the *National Codes,* is an alphanumeric coding system that uses a letter followed by four digits to identify products, supplies, and services that are not provided by physicians and other healthcare providers. These include ambulance services, prosthetics, and medical supplies used outside the healthcare provider's facility. The Center for Medicare & Medicaid Services (CMS), which is the federal agency that administers Medicare, Medicaid, the Health Insurance Portability and Accountability Act (HIPAA), and other healthcare programs, maintains Level II.

4. Current Procedural Terminology

In 1966, the AMA created the **CPT manual** (www.ama-assn.org/go/cpt) as a tool for reporting procedures and services. Four years later the CPT grew into three editions, referred to as sections and called *Categories I, II, and III.* In 1983, the CMS incorporated the CPT into the HCPCS to form a uniform system of reporting procedures and services for billing purposes.

Category I contains codes approved by the CPT editorial panel of the AMA and includes the majority of codes. This category is further grouped into sections based on medical specialties such as surgery, and within these sections are procedures and services, such as a biopsy. Any physician might be able to perform a procedure or service even though her practice might seem outside the specialty. For example, a dermatologist can perform an incision and drainage of an abscess, which is a procedure listed in the surgery section of Category I.

Category II contains optional measures used to treat a patient such as tracking the patient's blood pressure, weight management, or tobacco intervention. Category II items are not used for payment because they are part of the physician's normal evaluation and management of the patient, which is a Category I procedure.

Category II is divided into sections each with its own numbering system such as

- Diagnostic and screening processes or results
- Therapeutic, preventive, or other interventions
- Follow-up or other outcomes and patient safety

Category III contains temporary codes used to describe emerging technology, services, and procedures that have not been approved by the Food and Drug Administration (FDA) or not regularly performed by healthcare providers. Category III is used for collecting information about those procedures and services rather than for billing. Codes for this category are found following the medicine section of the CPT.

5. Inside the CPT Manual

The CPT manual has six sections, each having a range of codes:

- Evaluation and management 99201–99499
- Anesthesia 00100–01999, 99100–99140
- Surgery 10021–69990
- Radiology 70010–79999
- Pathology and laboratory 80048–89356
- Medicine 90281–99199, 99500–99600

The first digits indicate the section. For example, anesthesia codes begin with 0 and surgery codes begin with 1 through 6. This means that surgery has six sections. Each section has its own set of billing rules.

At the beginning of each section of the CPT manual are guidelines helpful to a medical insurance specialist. It contains information such as definitions, unlisted services, clinical examples, and tips to make it easy to code.

Sections are divided into subsections, subheadings, categories, and subcategories under which are the related procedures and services. Descriptions of procedures and services are listed alphabetically followed by the CPT code.

There are two types of CPT codes: stand-alone and indented. A **stand-alone code** specifies a procedure or service. A semicolon will follow a stand-alone procedure if an indented code is also available. The semicolon will indicate alternative body sites, procedures, or an extent of service. An **indented code** modifies the procedure or service. For example, 27846 is a stand-alone code for the open treatment of an ankle dislocation, with or without percutaneous skeletal fixation; without repair or internal fixation. 27848 is an indented code that specifies that the open treatment of an ankle dislocation was performed with repair or internal or external fixation. An indented code appears beneath the related stand-alone code in the CPT manual.

CPT Two-Digit Modifier

A **two-digit modifier** can be placed at the end of the code to indicate that something unusual occurred. Let's say that two surgeons performed the surgery that removed the mass from our patient. One was the primary surgeon and the other was the assisting surgeon. Halfway through the operation, the primary surgeon left the operating room and the assisting surgeon becomes primary.

Each surgeon uses the CPT code to bill for the procedure and uses a modifier to indicate the surgeon's role in the procedure. For example, modifier -62 indicates a primary surgeon and modifier -80 indicates an assisting surgeon. Appendix A in the CPT manual lists all modifiers and explains how to use them.

Coding for Unlisted Procedures

Some procedures and services are listed in the CPT manual usually because they are unusual, experimental, or not widely performed by healthcare providers. At the end of each subsection or heading are codes that can be used for unlisted procedures. For example, a new cardiac surgery procedure is assigned 33999. The last two 9s indicate that this is an unlisted procedure of cardiac surgery. The first three digits indicate the subheading that relates to the unlisted procedure.

6. Level II National Codes

National codes are used for procedures and services that are not covered by CPT codes. These include procedures and services performed by dentists, orthodontists, and allied healthcare providers such as ambulance services.

All Medicare and Medicaid claims for non-CPT procedures and services must include a Level II code that identifies the procedure or service. Many third-party payers also require that a national code be used for non-Medicare and non-Medicaid patients to ensure a uniform system for gathering healthcare data and for billing.

A Level II code (Table 5–1) consists of a letter (except V, W, X, Y, and Z) followed by four numbers. Letters K, G, Q, and S indicate temporary assignment of a procedure or service. For example, K is used for durable medical equipment that hasn't been assigned a permanent letter, and G is the temporary code for procedures and professional services. Temporary procedures and professional services are usually given a permanent letter when the Level II list is updated annually by the CMS.

Level II codes are used for outpatient services and for certain physicians that administer medication which utilize the J codes found in the HCPCS manual.

TABLE 5–1 Descriptions of First Letters of National Codes

National Code Group	Description
A	Transportation services, including ambulance medical and surgical supplies Administrative, miscellaneous, and investigational
B	Enteral and parenteral therapy
C	Temporary hospital OPPS
D	Dental procedures
E	Durable medical equipment
G	Temporary (procedures/professional services)
J	Drugs administered other than oral method
K	Temporary (durable medical equipment)
L	Orthotics and prosthetics
M	Medical services
P	Pathology and laboratory services
Q	Temporary (procedures, services, and supplies)
R	Diagnostic radiology services
S	Temporary National Codes (developed by BC/BS)
T	State Medicaid agencies
V	Vision services

Abbreviations: BC/BS, Blue Cross/Blue Shield; OPPS, outpatient prospective payment system.

Healthcare facilities use the diagnosis from **ICD-10-CM** and utilize ICD-10-CM, and Volume 3 to code claims. Level II codes are located in the HCPCS manual.

7. ICD-10-CM

The International Statistical Classification of Diseases and Related Health Problems (ICD) is the coding system developed by the World Health Organization and used to record diagnosis, treatments, and other information about patients. Versions of the coding system are identified by a number.

The National Center for Health Statistics in the United States created a modified version of ICD-10 referred to as *Clinical Modification* (ICD-10-CM). The CMS created a procedure coding system commonly referred to as *ICD-10-PCS.*

Healthcare has changed dramatically since ICD-9-CM was implemented nearly 25 years ago. There are new treatments, new medical devices, and newly identified disorders that have made the ICD-9-CM coding system inefficient. In addition, insurers, government agencies, healthcare providers, and others in the healthcare industry need an ever-growing amount of information to properly manage their aspect of the healthcare industry. ICD-9-CM is limited and could not facilitate the demand for information.

ICD-10-CM increases the amount of available diagnosis code. ICD-9-CM uses a five-position alphanumeric code that can generate 13,000 diagnosis codes. ICD-10-CM consists of seven-position numeric code that can generate 68,000 diagnosis codes. The additional codes enable more information to be conveyed in a code.

In addition, consistent terminology is now used throughout the ICD-10-CM and codes can be combined to reduce the number of codes that are needed to report the patient's complete condition. There are many subtle changes that make coding more efficient. For example, anatomical references are made as right arm or right leg.

Moving from ICD-9-CM to ICD-10-CM is not straightforward because ICD-9-CM codes don't map to ICD-10-CM directly. ICD-10-CM provides additional codes to increase the information that can be coded; therefore one ICD-9-CM code may expand into many ICD-10-CM codes making mapping to ICD-10-CM impossible.

CODING ALERT

ICD-9-CM codes, referred to as a *legacy coding system,* will be used as archive data but not support for new data.

ICD-10-CM has a chronological list of codes within 21 chapters that represents diseases and injuries. Chapters are based on the body systems or conditions. ICD-10-CM codes are displayed within code blocks sometimes referred to as *major topic headings.* Code blocks are divided into groups that are identified by a three-character disease category such as Intestinal Infectious Diseases, A00-A09.

All categories contain a three-character identifier. Subcategories contain either a four, five, or six character code. The final subdivision is an extension digit. An ICD- 10-CM code can have three, four, five, six, or seven characters.

There is a placeholder character used for the fifth character in some six-character codes. The placeholder character is an "x" and is used to perform future expansion. For example, H62.8x1 is such a code. The x must be present; otherwise the code is invalid.

Categories that contain seven characters must have codes of seven characters. If the code is less than seven characters then an x must be placed as the seventh character.

Z codes are used to describe factors influencing health status and contact with the health services and are located in Chapter 21 of ICD-10-CM. Z codes are reported as diagnosis codes because some classify situations associated with the procedure such as a canceled procedure. Don't use Z codes to report a procedure.

CODING ALERT

An external cause code is used to report events that caused the disorder such as accidents and assaults. External cause codes do not influence reimbursement except reporting it will expedite the claim since it explains the circumstances surrounding the treatment. External cause codes are in Chapters 19 and 20 of ICD-10-CM.

Morphology Codes

Morphology is the description of a type of neoplasm. Neoplasm is an abnormal growth of tissue that may or may not be cancer. Neoplasm is not reported on a claim but is reported to the state cancer registries using ICD-10-CM.

A neoplasm is a new tumor caused by out of control reproduction of cells. Chapter 2 of ICD-10-CM classifies neoplasm by site referred to as *topography* and not by type of cell. Chapter 13 contains codes for diseases of connective tissues.

Morphology codes begin with the letter M and are followed by five digits ranging from M8000/0 to M9989/3. The digit after the slash is referred to as a *behavior code* that indicates if the tumor is malignant, benign, within the original site (in situ), or is uncertain. Table 5–2 contains a listing of diagnostic coding guidelines section. These guidelines are used for reporting practitioner office visits.

TABLE 5–2 ICD-10-CM Diagnosis Coding Sections and Related Descriptions

	Section	Description
A	Selected of first-listed condition	The diagnosis, condition, problem, or other reasons for the visit to an outpatient setting. Two or more visits may be required before a diagnosis is confirmed. Outpatient includes hospital observation status for not more than 23 h and 59 min; hospital clinic, emergency department, same-day surgery of not more than 23 h and 59 min; or ambulatory surgery center.
B	List of diseases (A00-T88, Z00-Z99)	This must be used to identify diagnoses, symptoms, conditions, problems, complaints, or other reason for the encounter.
C	Diagnosis codes	The diagnosis code describes the patient's condition including symptoms, problems, or reasons for the encounter. In outpatient surgery, the first-listed diagnosis is the reason for the surgery even if the surgery is cancelled. In the observation stay, the first-listed diagnosis is the medical condition being observed. If the patient develops a complication, then the complication is the second-listed diagnosis.
D	Signs and symptoms	The signs and symptoms code identifies signs and symptoms identified by the practitioner. These are used when a diagnosis has not been established or confirmed.
E	Encounters for circumstances other than a disease or injury	These codes are used to describe encounters such as observation following a motor vehicle accident. The patient does not report any complaint and the practitioner doesn't find any physical signs of injury.
F	Detail codes	This lists a full description of the encounter.
G	Diagnosis, condition, problem, or other reason for the encounter	This code is used to report any coexisting conditions that were medically managed or that influenced treatment during the encounter.
H	Uncertain diagnoses	Avoid coding a diagnosis as questionable or working diagnosis. Uncertain diagnoses also referred to as *qualified diagnoses* are commonly used for hospital inpatient admissions. Instead of reporting an uncertainty, use a code that indicates the highest degree of certainty of a diagnosis for the encounter.

(Continued)

TABLE 5–2 ICD-10-CM Diagnosis Coding Sections and Related Descriptions (*Continued*)

	Section	Description
I	Chronic diseases	The chronic diseases code is used to indicate ongoing treatment.
J	Code all documented conditions that coexist	Code conditions that exist at the time of the encounter and not previously treated condition. History codes can be used as secondary codes to report previous conditions and family history that may impact the patient's current care and treatment.
K	Patient receiving diagnostic services only	This code is used when the patient encounter is for diagnostic services only. Enter the first-listed diagnosis. Chronic conditions may be reported as additional diagnoses.
L	Patients receiving therapeutic services only	This code is used when the patient receives therapeutic services only during the encounter.
M	Patients receiving preoperative evaluations only	This code is used when the encounter is for a preoperative evaluation only.
N	Ambulatory surgery	This code is used to identify the diagnosis related to the surgery. Use the postoperative diagnosis if it differs from the preoperative diagnosis.
O	Outpatient prenatal visits	This code is used for routine outpatient prenatal visits where no complications are present.
P	Encounters for general medical examinations with abnormal findings	This code is used for general examination without complications. An abnormal finding is listed as the first-listed diagnosis. Other abnormal findings are listed as secondary codes.

Encounters for Routine Health Screenings

A *screening* is a medical test given to a healthy person to detect early signs of a disease based on signs and symptoms identified by the practitioner. Tests rule out or confirm that the person has a disorder. Signs and symptoms are used to explain the reason why the practitioner ordered the test. The screening code is the first-listed code if the encounter is to screen for the disorder. That is, the person came to the practitioner to rule out a specific condition.

However, the screening code can be used as an additional code if the practitioner screens for the potential problem during a different encounter. For example, the person arrived with a sore throat and the practitioner discovered a lump on the person's leg, which has nothing to do with a sore throat. A screening code is not required if the screening is part of a routine examination such as a Pap smear during a routine pelvic examination. If a condition is discovered during the screen, then use an additional diagnosis code for the encounter.

> ### ⁰CODING ALERT
>
> Use the Z codes to report preoperative examination and pre-procedure tests used to clear the patient for surgery or a procedure but not if treatment is provided during those encounters.

The Z code is used to indicate that the screening was planned and a procedure code is used to indicate that the screening was performed. Z codes are used to describe routine examinations or administrative examinations such as a pre-employment physical. Additional codes such as those for history, preexisting conditions, and chronic conditions can also be used for administrative examinations that do not focus on a specific condition.

> ### CODING ALERT
>
> ICD-10-CM has codes that are used to distinguish between with and without normal findings known at the time of an encounter. There are specific codes used to identify specific abnormal findings. Assign the code for without abnormal findings if the examination showed abnormal findings but test results have yet to be received by the practitioner.

8. Hands-On Coding

Let's return to our patient who underwent surgery at the beginning of this chapter and identify the codes needed for this patient's medical insurance claim. Our first step is to identify the procedures and services for the patient. You'll find this information in the patient's folder given to you by the healthcare provider.

Not all procedures and services are chargeable to the insurer. You must decide which are chargeable based on your knowledge of the insurer's policies. For example, the initial claim to Medicare for a patient's surgery also includes a specific number of days of follow-up care. The follow-up visits are not chargeable.

Once you have identified the procedure and services that are chargeable, then you'll need to look up the corresponding code in the appropriate coding system. For example, Medicare and other government-sponsored programs require both HCPCS and CPT codes.

Look up the procedure or service in the index of the coding manual. The index of the HCPCS manual lists categories of procedures and services each having subcategories. A subcategory lists procedures and services and the corresponding codes. Avoid coding directly from the index. Instead, turn to the related page and make sure the description of the procedure or service is the same as the one you are billing.

Sometimes the healthcare provider uses synonyms, eponyms, or abbreviations rather than the full name that appears in the index. This means you'll need to ask the healthcare provider to clarify the name of the procedure or service before coding it.

A medication is identified by its generic name and dosages. However, many times the healthcare provider uses the drug's trade name instead. The index also contains the trade name for the medication and refers you to the generic name in the index rather than to the page of the manual that contains the generic medication. Consult a drug reference such as the **Physicians' Desk Reference** (PDR) if you are in doubt about a medication or dose.

Review the page in the manual that corresponds to the code to make sure that the description of the procedure or service in the manual is the same as that the healthcare provider performed. Determine if you need to add a modifier to the code by reviewing the available modifiers for each code that you selected.

On the claims form, list the date, the code, and the charge for each procedure or service. Place them in date order and then in rate order within each date with the highest rated procedure or service first as follows:

- Date of Procedure
  - 11/17/2001 99204
  - 11/20/2001 43215
  - 11/20/2001 74235
- Charge
  - $202
  - $355
  - $ 75

CASE STUDY

CASE 1

A 53-year-old woman who has employer-based health insurance was taken to the hospital for pain in the upper right area of her chest by ambulance. She underwent surgery to remove her gallbladder. The surgeon had to use an unusual treatment for this patient.

QUESTION 1. Why must the national codes be used for the claim?
ANSWER: Many third-party payers also require that a national code be used for non-Medicare and non-Medicaid patients to ensure a uniform system for gathering healthcare data and for billing.

QUESTION 2. Where would you find the modifier that indicates something unusual occurred?
ANSWER: Appendix A in the CPT manual lists all modifiers and explains how to use them.

QUESTION 3. What code range from the CPT manual would you use for a surgery procedure?
ANSWER: Surgery 10021–69990

QUESTION 4. Where would you find the unique code for procedures so you can submit a claim for reimbursement?
ANSWER: Healthcare Common Procedure Coding System (HCPCS)

FINAL CHECKUP

1. **What is HCPCS?**
   A. Healthcare Consistent Processing Coding System
   B. Healthcare Common Processing Coding System
   C. Healthcare Common Procedure Coding System
   D. Healthcare Consistent Procedure Coding System

2. **What does the National Code contain?**
   A. HCPCS Level II
   B. HCPCS Level III
   C. HCPCS Level IV
   D. HCPCS Level V

3. **What is the purpose of the Current Procedural Terminology Manual?**

   A. To help the physician reach a medical diagnosis

   B. To increase reimbursements from health insurers

   C. To prevent the medical billing specialists from making errors

   D. For reporting procedures and services

4. **What is represented by the first digits in the CPT manual?**

   A. The primary diagnosis

   B. The primary practitioner

   C. The practitioner

   D. The section of the manual

5. **A stand-alone code specifies a procedure or service.**

   A. True

   B. False

6. **An indented code modifies the procedure or service.**

   A. True

   B. False

7. **What is the purpose of a two-digit modifier?**

   A. Indicates that something usual occurred.

   B. Indicates that something unusual occurred.

   C. Indicates that the procedure was successful.

   D. Indicates that the procedure was performed in a hospital.

8. **You cannot code an experimental procedure.**

   A. True

   B. False

9. **National codes are used for procedures and services that are not covered by CPT codes.**

   A. True

   B. False

10. **You should refer to the Physicians' Desk Reference or similar publications when in doubt of the medication dose used in a procedure.**

    A. True

    B. False

CORRECT ANSWERS AND RATIONALES

1. C. Healthcare Common Procedure Coding System.
2. A. HCPCS Level II.
3. D. For reporting procedures and services.
4. D. The section of the manual.
5. A. True.
6. A. True.
7. B. Indicates that something unusual occurred.
8. B. False.
9. A. True.
10. A. True.

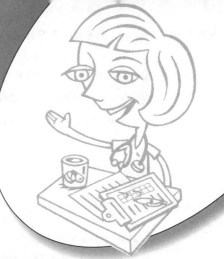

chapter 6

Introduction to Insurance Plans

LEARNING OBJECTIVES

14 Disability Insurance

15 Workers' Compensation

16 Liability Insurance and Healthcare

KEY TERMS

Exclusive Provider Organization (EPO)   Point of Service
Health Maintenance Organization   Preferred Provider Organization
Integrated Delivery System (IDS)   Triple Option Plans
Out-of-Pocket Maximum and Lifetime
  Payouts

1. What Is Insurance?

Healthcare providers will look toward you in your new role as a medical insurance specialist to guide them through the maze of health insurance plans to ensure that a steady stream of reimbursements flow into the practice. You must be knowledgeable about various kinds of healthcare plans and what each covers and how the plans protect patients from financial losses if they come down with an illness or get injured in an accident.

Insurance is a contract between two parties called an *insurance policy*. One party to the contract, called the *insured*, is at a potential financial loss from the possibility that certain events will occur. The other party, called an *insurer*, agrees to cover this financial loss in exchange for ongoing payments of money called a *premium*. The amount of the premium corresponds to the risk that the event will occur.

The insurer is betting that the event won't happen or if it does happen, the premiums paid prior to the event will cover the financial loss. Insurers hedge this bet by specifying inclusions, conditions, and exclusions in the contract. An *inclusion* is an event that the insurer will reimburse the insured if there is any financial loss related to the event. A *condition* is a set of circumstances in which the insurer will reimburse the insured if an inclusion occurs. An *exclusion* is an event not covered by the insurance policy.

For example, a person is at risk of being ill, which exposes her to medical expenses to restore her health. She could afford to pay for minor illnesses such as a sore throat, but a major illness would bankrupt her, so she purchases medical insurance from an insurer.

The insurer is financially exposed to the same risk as the insured. The insurer must be prepared to pay substantial money if the insured is afflicted with a major illness. However, the insurer uses a strategy to minimize this risk.

First, the insurer estimates the type of illnesses that might afflict a person based on his personal profile and the likelihood that it will occur. For example, a 20-year-old healthy man who is active could develop Type II diabetes during the year, but probably won't. A 53-year-old man who is 150 pounds overweight and works at a sedentary job could also develop Type II diabetes during the year—and there is a high probability that he will.

The insurer also estimates the cost of caring for illnesses that the person is likely to experience during the year. This enables the insurer to project reimbursement costs if he agrees to insure the person. These estimates also become the basis for setting the premium.

Next, those likely illnesses are listed as inclusions in the insurance policy. That is, the insurer is saying, "I will cover the cost of these illnesses."

Next, conditions are specified when the inclusions are reimbursed. A condition might state that the insurer will not reimburse the person for illnesses that result from a person exposing herself to risky situations such as skydiving and race car driving. Another condition might cap reimbursement at a fixed dollar amount.

And finally the insurer includes exclusions to exclude illnesses that were not part of its original estimate or are simply too costly to cover. For example, illnesses that occur due to an auto accident are excluded from coverage because these are covered by an auto insurance policy. However, the medical insurance might cover costs not covered by the auto insurer.

2. Sharing Risk

The insurer calculates the odds that over the insured period—usually 12 months—premiums received from the insured would be more than the insured is reimbursed for financial losses. This is the same type of calculation professional gamblers make when deciding whether or not to place a bet.

Calculations are based on the probability that the insured condition will occur during the insured period. In other words, what are the chances that the insured will contract an illness that is specified in the inclusion clause of the insurance policy and within terms set in the condition clause?

Probability is a mathematical guess based on statistics that measures the event. However, it is still a guess, which means there is a chance—a small one—that the person will experience an illness that will be expensive to treat. This is the risk the insurer bets won't happen.

The insurer protects himself from the chance of paying a greater than expected reimbursement in two ways. First, the insurer insures a group of people rather than individuals, and second, he purchases an insurance policy called *reinsurance*.

Insuring a group of people enables the insurer to spread the risk among more than one insured. A group typically consists of employees from the same employer, ranging in age from 18 to 60 years. Each pays a monthly premium based on the profile of the group. In total, these premiums should be sufficient to reimburse any illness covered by the group medical policy.

A reinsurance policy is a contract between an insurer and a reinsurer where the reinsurer agrees to cover financial losses of the insurer under specified inclusions, conditions, and exclusions in return for ongoing premiums.

3. How Insurers Make Money

Insurers make money by carefully investing premiums and by making more winning than losing bets. Each month the insurer estimates three amounts: revenue from premiums, reimbursements, and excess cash. Excess cash is the difference between the premiums and reimbursements. Excess cash is then reinvested, which generates additional revenue for the insurer.

Let's say that an insured paid a monthly premium of $500 to $6,000 for the entire year—and didn't file any claims. The insurer kept the $6,000, plus invested it during the year. If the investment returned 10%, then the insurer made an additional $600 above the premium.

Insurers expect to make reimbursements; however, they also take steps to minimize reimbursements by negotiating fees with healthcare providers and by establishing rules for reimbursements based on standard medical practices. For example, most practitioners diagnose a particular illness based on four laboratory tests. The insurer will refuse to pay for a fifth laboratory test unless the healthcare provider gives an acceptable medical rationale for the additional test.

Likewise, the insurer reduces reimbursements by encouraging the insured to care for him by going for routine examinations by a practitioner. Some illnesses are less costly to treat if caught at an early onset.

4. How Practitioners Make Money

Practitioners are paid in one of two ways depending on their practice—by salary if they are an employee of a healthcare facility or by procedure. In either case, insurer reimbursements are at a fixed-fee rate based on the procedure performed by the practitioner.

In some situations, a practitioner who joins a group practice is given a guaranteed salary in a relatively short period of time such as 3 years. After that period, the practitioner is paid according to procedures he/she performs.

Although practitioners set their own fees, they also negotiate lower fees with insurers. As a result, a practitioner might deal with 24 insurers, each setting a different reimbursement fee for hundreds of commonly performed procedures.

An insurer's fee schedule is based on negotiations with the healthcare provider and on the usual, customary, and reasonable fees that other practitioners within the area charged patients. Schedules get quickly outdated because new technology alters the way procedures are performed. For example, cataract surgery took up to 4 hours in 1985. Nowadays this operation takes 30 minutes. However, practitioners were still being reimbursed for 4 hours of work.

In order to rectify this problem, Harvard economist William Hsiao was hired by the federal government to create a better way to pay practitioners. He analyzed the practices of several thousand practitioners and devised a new reimbursement system that considers the practitioner's time, mental effort, technical skill, practitioner effort, judgment, and stress.

As a result, Hsiao developed a relative value for everything performed by a practitioner. Based on his study, the resource-based relative value scale (RBRVS) was developed for Medicare reimbursements. Medical procedures are ranked according to the relative cost to perform the procedure and then assigned three resource-based relative value units (RBRVUs): for practitioner's work, practice expense, and professional liability insurance. The sum of these RBRVUs is multiplied by a dollar conversion factor to derive the reimbursement fee. Private insurers adopted a similar plan that used its own multiplier factor.

Reimbursement fees are revenue—not profit—for a practitioner. The practitioner has to deduct expenses from the reimbursement fees. Depending on the practice, $100,000 is needed for office and clinical space, another $40,000 for malpractice insurance, plus additional amounts for the healthcare team and equipment. And if the practitioner is a surgeon, he has to pay nearly a quarter of the reimbursement to the surgery department of the healthcare facility.

Sometimes reimbursements are used to offset the cost of treating patients who do not have healthcare insurance. Ten percent of patients might fall into this category. Occasionally the claims are rejected by the insurer resulting in no payment for caring for a patient.

There can easily be situations when reimbursements are lower than expenses meaning that the practitioner loses money. Practitioners minimize this by screening new patients before making an appointment to ensure that they are covered by insurance and that the practitioner has a relationship with the insurer. They also make sure all the details are in order such as a referral number from the patient's primary-care practitioner. The referral number is included on the claim indicating the insurer that the patient has seen her primary-care practitioner before the visit. Failure to include this number could result in the claim being rejected by the insurer.

Practitioners are at the mercy of insurers who dictate the fees for each procedure. Practitioners increase their income by performing additional procedures. However, a few practitioners are able to set their own rates and bring in a substantial income from their practice by not accepting insurance. Patients pay cash and then submit the claim to their insurer for reimbursement. These fees are much higher than those set by insurers. Therefore, reimbursements don't cover the entire fee. For example, a surgeon might charge $8,000 for a gallbladder removal and the insurer reimburses the patient $800. In this case, the patient pays $8,000 and then pockets the $800 reimbursement.

5. Healthcare Financing

Healthcare insurance is a way to finance healthcare because it does not just insure for events that may not occur. For example, people buy automobile insurance but may go a lifetime without a car accident. But it is more than likely that everyone will get ill at some time. Depending on the type of healthcare insurance you have, it may also cover preventive care.

Healthcare insurance has evolved from benefits employers offered during World War II to entice employees to join their firm (see Chapter 1). Since then, it has become the de facto method of financing healthcare.

Employers are expected to provide healthcare benefits to employees, and the federal government provides the same for the elderly and disabled (Medicare) and the poor (Medicaid).

However, the spiraling cost of healthcare has priced healthcare insurance beyond the reach of many small businesses. Furthermore, people who have chronic illnesses and those in high-risk categories find individual healthcare premiums unaffordable. For example, a 62-year-old retiree might be expected to pay $8,000 a year for health insurance until he reaches 65 when he qualifies for Medicare.

Since health insurance premiums are based on the health profile of a group, such as employees of a firm, some employers carefully—and quietly—hire employees who are likely to have a low medical risk. These are typically younger, healthy people.

As a result, a third of the people in the United States are priced out of health-care insurance forcing them to go without medical coverage. And those with medical coverage expect to pay more out-of-pocket expenses in the form of deductibles and other fees.

The financial costs of healthcare cause many uninsured people to avoid medical care until their health condition is no longer tolerable at which point they visit an emergency room. Their condition worsened to a point where only expensive medical procedures could restore their health. The healthcare facility absorbs this expense and then passes it along as higher medical fees to those who are insured.

6. Health Insurance Premium

An insurance premium is the amount that the insured pays to the insurer to cover her medical expenses based on the terms of the policy. Premiums are paid monthly, quarterly, or annually. Employers may deduct a portion of the premium from an employee's paycheck and then pay the insurer at the end of the month.

A premium isn't allocated to pay an insured's medical expense directly. Instead it is pooled with other premiums and used to pay claims for all those who the insurer insures.

Besides all or part of a premium, depending upon the type of insurance coverage, the insured is also expected to pay the cost of a deductible, co-payment, and coinsurance. A deductible is the amount the insured pays for healthcare before the insurer pays. Let's say a person has a $1,000 deductible. He is expected to pay the first $1,000 of medical care out-of-pocket; afterward the insurer pays.

A deductible extends for a year beginning at the start of the policy. This means that each year the person must pay the first $1,000 of medical care if she has a $1,000 deductible. The amount of the deductible affects the premium cost. Typically, a higher deductible results in a lower premium.

A co-payment is a dollar amount that the insured is required to pay directly to the healthcare provider for each visit. The co-payment is in addition to the deductible. The amount of the co-payment affects the premium cost. A higher co-payment usually results in a lower premium.

Coinsurance is a percentage of the total medical costs divided between the insured and the insurer. In an 80/20 coinsurance, the patient pays 20% and the insurer pays 80% of the allowed charges.

Out-of-Pocket Maximum and Lifetime Payouts

The out-of-pocket maximum is a provision in a healthcare insurance policy that limits the amount that the insured pays in a year for medical expenses. This protects the insured from paying too much excess in addition to the premium. After the limit is reached, the insurer pays medical expenses at 100%.

Formerly, insurers could protect themselves from paying excess for an insured's medical care by implementing a lifetime payout provision. This provision sets a limit on the amount the insurer is responsible to pay for the insured's medical care for the insured's entire lifetime. However, the Affordable Care Act prohibits health plans from establishing a lifetime dollar limit on most benefits. The Affordable Care Act restricts do away with annual dollar limits.

However, lifetime limits and yearly limits can apply to healthcare services that are not considered essential health benefits. Essential healthcare services include

- Ambulatory patient services.
- Emergency services.
- Hospitalization.
- Pregnancy, maternity, and newborn care before and after birth.
- Mental health and substance-use disorder services, including counseling and psychotherapy.
- Prescription drugs.
- Rehabilitative and devices. These are services and devices to help people with injuries, disabilities, or chronic conditions recover skills.
- Laboratory services.
- Preventive and wellness case.
- Chronic disease management.
- Pediatric care.

7. Medical Coverage

Healthcare coverage is generally divided into basic coverage and extra coverage. Basic coverage includes preventative care, diagnostic tests, hospital care, extended care, emergency care, home healthcare, and prescription drugs. Extra coverage includes dental care, vision care, drug and alcohol abuse treatment, chiropractic care, and mental healthcare.

The type of coverage a person receives depends on her needs and the affordability of the premium. A broader coverage increases the premium cost. Some people forgo extra coverage in order to keep the premium affordable.

When choosing a policy, the insured

- Selects a policy that has basic medical coverage because this covers the most common medical care needed during the year.

- Uses his family history to determine the likelihood that he'll experience illnesses that are beyond basic medical coverage. For instance, he might be at risk for an inherited disease that requires more intense treatment than is covered under a basic medical insurance policy.

- Forecasts his future medical needs. If he expects to marry and have children, then it is best to look for a policy that covers his spouse, maternity care, and children.

8. Assessing the Value of a Healthcare Policy

Many people ask, "Is healthcare insurance worth the premium?" To answer this question for yourself, you first must estimate your healthcare expenses without medical coverage. This is tricky because you must forecast when you are going to be ill and the nature of your illness.

Begin the assessment by looking at the past and review your medical history. Some people rarely fall ill beyond an annual head cold and therefore almost never visit a practitioner. Others experience chronic illnesses that require frequent practitioner visits, medical tests, and possibly hospitalization followed by therapy.

Tally the expenses that would have been incurred if you didn't have medical insurance over the past 5 years. Your healthcare provider can give you fees that are charged to patients who don't have medical insurance.

Next, determine the types of illnesses that you are at risk of contracting. Although it seems like you need a crystal ball to do this, your healthcare provider can probably assist with this question. His response is based on your family medical history, your medical history, work environment, personal habits, and age. For example, someone who exercises frequently, eats properly, and has never smoked or drank alcohol is less likely to contract certain illnesses than someone who smokes, drinks, doesn't exercise, and eats junk food.

Once future illnesses are identified, determine the annual medical cost of caring for those illnesses. Be sure to adjust these figures to reflect the annual increase in fees. Your healthcare provider can assist with this assessment.

With the actual and projected cost of your healthcare at hand, compare them to annual premiums to determine if a policy makes economic sense. Be sure to consider the out-of-pocket expenses that you'll have, such as monthly premium cost, deductible, co-payment, and the lifetime payout provision.

Medical coverage in the United States is generally considered an all-or-nothing situation. That is, people expect the medical insurer to pay for all medical expenses; otherwise they forgo coverage. However, medical coverage is adjustable based on how much coverage a person requires.

For example, a person in good health might decide on a policy that has a relatively high deductible because she is rarely ill. The policy covers extraordinary expenses that probably won't—but could—arise.

By adjusting the co-payment, deductible, and types of coverage, the insured can find an economic balance between costs and benefits.

9. Types of Healthcare Plans

Health insurance policies fall into three general categories: managed care health plans; indemnity healthcare plans, which are also referred to as *fee-for-service health plans*; and plans that combine both. Each category has a different approach to healthcare.

1. Managed care plans
   - Focus on maintaining good health and lowering the risk of developing more severe illnesses—and as a result lowering cost.
   - Require the insured choose a healthcare provider from an approved list; otherwise the insurer won't reimburse medical costs.
   - May have a deductible depending on the model.
   - Cover preventative care.
   - Are less flexible than indemnity healthcare plans when choosing a healthcare provider.

- Are easier for the insurer to predict healthcare costs.
2. Indemnity healthcare plans
    - Focus on treating current illnesses.
    - Allow the insured to choose the healthcare provider.
    - Require the insured pay the healthcare provider and then submit a claim to the insurer for reimbursement. Today many people authorize their healthcare provider to submit claims directly to and be reimbursed by the insurer.
    - Have greater flexibility in choice of healthcare providers.
    - May not cover preventative care such as practitioner examinations and vaccinations.
    - Do not count out-of-pocket expenses for preventative care toward the deductible.
    - Make it harder for the insurer to predict healthcare costs.
3. Combined plans
    - Combine features of managed care and indemnity healthcare plans.
    - Allow the insured to choose to receive care from approved or unapproved healthcare providers.
    - Have a lower out-of-pocket cost for the insured if treated by an approved healthcare provider.
    - Have a higher out-of-pocket cost for the insured if treated by an unapproved healthcare provider.

10. Types of Indemnity Insurance

There are three types of indemnity insurance: basic health insurance, major medical insurance, and comprehensive insurance.

- Basic health insurance covers hospital care including room and board along with X-rays, medicine, and other similar hospital services. Also covered are visits to healthcare providers and surgery.
- Major medical insurance includes treatment for costly illnesses and extensive coverage for hospital costs.
- Comprehensive insurance combines both basic healthcare and major medical insurance coverage.

11. Types of Managed Care Plans

There are six managed care models: Exclusive Provider Organization (EPO), Integrated Delivery System (IDS), triple option plan, preferred provider organizations (PPO), point-of-service (POS), and health maintenance organizations (HMOs). All have a network of healthcare providers that if used will lower out-of-pocket expenses.

Exclusive Provider Organization

An EPO is a network of healthcare providers who have contracts with specific health insurers. Policyholders are required to select a primary-care practitioner who is a member of the EPO. The primary-care practitioner provides preventative care, primary care, and refers the policyholder to a specialist when necessary. The specialist is also a member of the EPO. The policyholder is able to choose a practitioner who does not belong to the EPO; however, the policyholder's out-of-pocket expense is appreciably higher if the policyholder chooses a practitioner who is a member of the EPO. This is because out-of-network practitioners do not have a contract with the health insurer.

Integrated Delivery System

An IDS is an organization of healthcare providers who provides policyholders with a coordinated continued care. The IDS payment is based on achieving expected outcomes. Integrated services include preventive care, outpatient care, inpatient care, same-day surgery, home healthcare, social services, and rehabilitation care.

Triple Option Plans

Triple option plan, also called a *cafeteria plan* or *flexible benefit plan,* provides customers with a choice of a traditional health insurance plan, an HMO, and PPO. The goal of triple option plans is to cover adverse selection. **Adverse selection** is a group of customers who are sicker than the insured group called the *risk pool.*

Preferred Provider Organization

In a PPO-managed care plan, the insured can choose to go to a healthcare provider who is in-network or out-of-network. There is a higher out-of-pocket expense when going out-of-network. This means that the insured can consult any specialist without first having to see her primary-care practitioner. However, treatment and co-payments are more expensive than when going to an in-network practitioner. Furthermore, the insured might incur a high deductible.

PPO is the most expensive type of managed-care plan if the insured goes out-of-network frequently for care because reimbursements are based on reasonable and customary fees. Actual fees might be higher requiring the insured to pay the difference.

Point of Service

A POS-managed care plan requires the insured to choose a primary-care practitioner who is responsible for managing the insured healthcare. The primary-care practitioner must be with the POS network of healthcare providers.

Although the insured is not limited to in-network healthcare providers, the primary-care practitioner must make referrals to specialists. These specialists can be in-network or out-of-network. However, it is highly likely that an in-network specialist will be referred. As long as the insured stays within network, co-payments are relatively low and there isn't a deductible. For out-of-network care, the insured should expect high co-payments and a deductible.

Health Maintenance Organization

An HMO offers a variety of medical benefits, but some plans offer fewer services than others. The insured selects a primary-care practitioner from practitioners within the HMO who then is responsible for his healthcare, treatment approval, and referrals to specialists.

Except for emergencies, the insured must use healthcare providers and healthcare facilities that are part of the HMO. Care received outside the HMO that is not approved by the primary care practitioner isn't reimbursed.

There are times when an insured may wait longer for an appointment with a healthcare provider than with other types of managed care plans. Furthermore, it is more complicated to see a specialist in an HMO than in other plans because the primary-care practitioner must refer the insured to the specialist.

HMOs are less costly than other managed-care plans because there is a monthly premium and few other expenses if care is given by HMO healthcare providers. However, they are the most costly if most care is given by healthcare providers who are not part of the HMO.

12. Health Savings Accounts

Although a health savings account (HSA) isn't an insurance plan, it is a way for people to pay medical care in conjunction with a medical insurance policy. Regular deposits are made to an HSA using pretax dollars. A premium is paid for a medical insurance policy that has a high deductible and a relatively low premium.

Routine medical care expenses, such as office visits and prescriptions, are paid for by withdrawals from the HSA. Even the premium can be paid from the HSA. The medical insurance policy covers emergencies and major medical coverage. Funds not used remain in the HSA and draw tax-free interest until they are spent or until the person retires.

13. Auto Insurance and Healthcare

At first you may think that auto insurance has nothing to do with healthcare, but it has because auto insurance reimburses for accidental bodily injury and other medical expenses related to an automobile accident.

The liability protection of an auto insurance policy reimburses medical expenses of those injured in an accident caused by the insured. Many auto insurance policies also offer personal injury protection (PIP). PIP reimburses the insured for medical expenses regardless of who caused the accident.

When a person incurs medical expenses related to an automobile accident, the auto insurance policy is the primary insurance and the person's medical insurance is the secondary insurance. A primary insurer reimburses for expenses up to the limits specified in the policy. A secondary insurer reimburses expenses that exceed the limits of the primary insurance policy. Some states allow the insured to dictate which insurance will be primary, the PIP or the medical carrier. Check the laws in your state.

14. Disability Insurance

Disability insurance covers an employee for lost income and medical expenses resulting from illness or injury. A person must have been employed when the disability occurred and no longer be able to do customary work as defined in the disability insurance policy. The disability must be certified by a licensed healthcare provider, and the employee must remain under care until he is no longer disabled.

The healthcare provider must be careful to document treatment for the disability separately from treatment for other illnesses. Disability claims must not be confused with claims for the patient's other illnesses.

Patients can be ineligible for disability claims if they are receiving unemployment insurance benefits, become disabled while committing a felony, are in jail or a halfway house, or fail to let a healthcare provider verify the disability.

The healthcare provider who certifies the disability is required to estimate the date that the person will recover from the disability. Recertification is necessary if the patient is still disabled beyond this date.

15. Workers' Compensation

Workers' compensation is an insurance policy purchased by an employer who pays an employee's medical expenses for work-related injuries and diseases. The injury must have occurred as a result of employment.

For example, injuries a housepainter incurs by falling from a scaffold while painting a house for her employer are covered by workers' compensation. However, an employee who is a smoker and develops lung cancer isn't covered unless it is proven that he was exposed to the carcinogen that caused the cancer in his workplace.

Some injuries are referred to as a neutral risk and may or may not be covered by workers' compensation. For example, in the case of a teacher who is bitten by a stray dog while standing on the sidewalk supervising students boarding the school bus, a determination must be made whether or not this injury occurred because of her employment with the school district.

Workers' compensation insurance provides two categories of benefits. These are indemnity and medical benefits. Indemnity benefits compensate for lost income, and medical benefits reimburse for medical expenses.

16. Liability Insurance and Healthcare

Liability insurance covers financial losses that occur when a third party is injured by the insured. The third party is reimbursed for medical care among other losses. The liability policy is the primary insurance for healthcare reimbursement and the third party's medical insurance is the secondary insurance. The third party's medical insurer may reimburse for medical care if the liability insurance does not cover the medical expenses.

Medical claims are filed with the liability insurer using a patient's billing statement instead of a medical claims form. The billing statement is addressed to the liability insurer and must include the name of the policyholder and the liability policy number. If reimbursement is denied, then a medical claims form is submitted to the patient's health insurer along with a copy of the denial.

CASE STUDY

CASE 1

During an interview for a medical coding and billing position, the practice manager asks you the following questions about reimbursement. What is your best response?

QUESTION 1. What is the resource-based relative value scale (RBRVS)?
ANSWER: The RBRVS was developed for Medicare reimbursements. Medical procedures are ranked according to the relative cost to perform the procedure and then assigned three resource-based relative value units (RBRVUs): for practitioner's work, practice expense, and professional liability insurance. The sum of these RBRVUs is multiplied by a dollar conversion factor to derive the reimbursement fee. Private insurers adopted a similar plan that used its own multiplier factor.

QUESTION 2. Are reimbursement fees provided for the practice?
ANSWER: Reimbursement fees are revenue—not profit—for a practitioner. The practitioner has to deduct expenses from the reimbursement fees. Depending on the practice, $100,000 is needed for office and clinical space, another $40,000 for malpractice insurance, plus additional amounts for the healthcare team and equipment. And if the practitioner is a surgeon, he has to pay nearly a quarter of the reimbursement to the surgery department of the healthcare facility.

QUESTION 3. How are practitioners paid?
ANSWER: Practitioners are paid in one of two ways depending on their practice— by salary if they are employees of a healthcare facility or by procedure. In either case, insurer reimbursements are at a fixed-fee rate based on the procedure performed by the practitioner.

QUESTION 4. How do insurance companies calculate premiums?
ANSWER: The insurer calculates the odds that over the insured period—usually 12 months—premiums received from the insured would be more than the insured is reimbursed for financial losses. This is the same type of calculation professional gamblers make when deciding whether or not to place a bet.

FINAL CHECKUP

1. **How does an insurer spread the risk of high reimbursements?**
   A. Insuring a group of people
   B. Insuring individuals
   C. Insuring only groups of young people
   D. All of the above

2. **What does an insured pay to the insurer for healthcare coverage?**
   A. A down payment
   B. A reimbursement
   C. A premium
   D. None of the above

3. **Has a lifetime payout provision been eliminated from healthcare insurance?**
   A. Yes, by the Affordable Care Act.
   B. No, the Affordable Care Act prohibits exclusion of a lifetime payout clause.
   C. Yes, however, lifetime limits can apply to healthcare services that are not considered essential health benefits.
   D. Yes, except for all hospitalizations.

4. **The focus of managed-care plans is on maintaining good health and lowering the risk of developing more severe illness.**
   A. True
   B. False

5. **An exclusion is an event covered by the insurance policy.**
   A. True
   B. False

6. **A condition is**
   A. A group of practitioners in which the insurer will reimburse the insured if the practitioner cares for the insured.
   B. A set of circumstances in which the insurer will not reimburse the insured if an inclusion occurs.
   C. A set of circumstances in which the insurer will reimburse the insured if an inclusion occurs.
   D. A set of circumstances in which the insurer will reimburse the insured if an exclusion occurs.

7. **Indemnity healthcare plans focus on treating current illnesses.**
   A. True
   B. False

8. **How does a person determine if the healthcare insurance is worth the premium?**

    A. You first must estimate your healthcare expenses of your current illness.

    B. You first must estimate your healthcare expenses without medical coverage.

    C. You first must estimate your healthcare expenses of your all previous illness.

    D. You first must estimate your premium cost for your all previous illness.

9. **An exclusive provider organization (EPO) is a network of healthcare providers that have contracts with specific health insurers. Policyholders are required to select a primary-care practitioner who is a member of the EPO. The primary-care practitioner provides preventative care, primary care, and refers the policyholder to a specialist when necessary.**

    A. True

    B. False

10. **For an insured covered by a health maintenance organization (HMO), except for emergencies, the insured must use healthcare providers and healthcare facilities that are part of the HMO. Care received outside the HMO that is not approved by the primary-care practitioner isn't reimbursed.**

    A. True

    B. False

CORRECT ANSWERS AND RATIONALES

1. A. Insuring a group of people.
2. C. A premium.
3. C. Yes, however, lifetime limits can apply to healthcare services that are not considered essential health benefits.
4. A. True.
5. B. False.
6. C. A set of circumstances in which the insurer will reimburse the insured if an inclusion occurs.
7. A. True.
8. B. You first must estimate your healthcare expenses without medical coverage.
9. A. True.
10. A. True.

chapter 7

The Insurance Claim Cycle

KEY TERMS

Basic Insurance
Blue Cross and Blue Shield
CMS-1500 Data Elements
Exclusive Provider Organization
Government Insurance Plans
Health Maintenance Organizations
Health Savings Account Plan
HIPAA Data Elements
Integrated Delivery System

Major Medical Insurance
Managed-Care Models
Medicaid
Medicare
Point-of-Service Plan
Preferred Provider Organization
Triple Option Plan
Workers' Compensation Insurance

1. Inside the Insurance Claim Cycle

Pretend for a moment that you're a physician. You've finished caring for your patient. Now you want to get paid, but first you must file a claim with your patient's medical insurance company and wait for it to approve the claim—and wait for it to send you a reimbursement check.

Now multiply this scenario by 150–200 patients a day, which is a typical patient load for a group medical practice, and you'll understand why there is a demand for medical insurance specialists.

Processing medical claims is a mission-critical function for every physician practice, hospital, outpatient clinic, hospice, and laboratory. Any delay in processing directly impacts the bottom line because it delays payment.

The insurance claim cycle is a process that you follow to bill a third-party payer for a patient's medical care and to receive appropriate and timely payment. The cycle begins when the patient first arrives at the healthcare facility and is asked to provide information about medical insurance coverage.

Besides being asked to fill out a health questionnaire, the patient is asked to fill out a patient information form that is used to identify the patient's medical insurer and the patient's policy number. A policy number identifies the medical insurance plan that covers the patient's medical bills.

The patient is also asked to sign an assignment of benefit and release of information that is usually found at the bottom of the patient information form (Figure 7–1). By signing this form, the patient permits the healthcare provider to file a claim directly with the patient's medical insurer and allows the medical

Welcome

Please complete this form completely in ink. This information will remain confidential.

Patient Information

Last name:	First name:	Initial:	Date of birth:	Home phone:

Address:			Marital Status: (check appropriate box) ⑥ S ⑥ M ⑥ D W	Sex ⑥ M ⑥ F
City:	State:	Zip:	Social Security Number:	
Patient's employer: (If student, name of school.)			Employment address: Business phone:	
Bill to:			Relationship:	
Address:			City:	State: Zip:

NOTIFY IN CASE OF EMERGENCY

Name:	Relationship:
Address:	Phone:
City: State: Zip:	

INSURANCE INFORMATION

Primary insurance company:	Secondary insurance company:
Subscriber's name: DOB:	Subscriber's name: DOB:
Policy #: Group #:	Policy #: Group #:

OTHER INFORMATION

Reason for visit:	Name of referring physician:
_____ *Patient's signature/Parent or guardian's signature*	Today's date

FIGURE 7–1 · Patient information form.

insurer to reimburse the healthcare provider. Furthermore, it also authorizes the healthcare provider to share the patient's medical information with the medical insurer.

The last phase of this initial step is to make a copy of the patient's medical insurance card. The medical insurance card contains the patient's name, insurance policy and/or group number, and contact information for the medical insurance which is kept with the patient's insurance records.

2. Verify Insurance Information

Verification is the next step in the cycle. You must immediately verify that the policy is active, whether the patient requires a referral, the type of plan, and the deductible information if any to ensure the healthcare provider will be reimbursed for the patient's medical cost. Although the patient's medical insurance card identifies that the patient has medical coverage, it is insufficient verification because the policy might have lapsed.

There are ways in which to verify that a patient has medical coverage. For example, the medical insurer's Web site, by telephone, or through an insurance eligibility verification system, such as Emdeon or Passport. The patient's medical insurance card typically lists Web sites and phone numbers to use for verification. Some medical insurers provide a card reader to healthcare providers who are members of their healthcare provider network.

The medical insurer will tell you whether the patient's medical plan is active and who in the patient's family is covered under the policy. Some medical policies cover the patient's complete family, while others restrict coverage, such as covering the patient's child only through college or until the age of 26. It is important that you learn about these restrictions and that the patient is also aware of them before beginning medical treatment.

The medical insurer also tells you the types of treatment covered in the schedule of benefits. The schedule of benefits is a list of medical expenses that a health plan covers. The treatment that the patient needs may not be covered by the plan, and the reimbursement rate might be less than the healthcare provider's fee. In these situations the patient must make alternative arrangements to cover these expenses before treatment begins.

Perform the verification process upon each patient's visit to ensure that the patient's eligibility hasn't changed.

Sometimes a patient is covered by more than one medical insurance policy. For example, the patient's employer and his spouse's employer both provide family medical coverage. In this situation, verify both insurance policies and ask each medical insurer which policy is primary. The claim is made against the primary policy first. If the reimbursement doesn't cover the full fee, then the claim is made against the secondary policy for the difference.

Medical insurers determine the primary policy by following these rules:

- The patient's employer-provided policy is the primary policy and the spouse's employer-provided policy is the secondary policy.

- If the patient has two jobs and each employer provides medical coverage, then the policy that is in effect the longest is the primary policy.

- If the patient is a child who lives with both parents and is covered by two medical policies—provided by each parent's employer—primary coverage is provided by the employer of the parent whose birthday comes first in the calendar year. If both parents have the same birthday (different years), then the policy that has been in effect longer is the primary policy.

- If the patient is a child of divorced parents and is covered by policies provided by both parent's employers, then the custodial parent's insurance is primary.

- If the parent remarries, then the custodial stepparent's plan becomes secondary and the noncustodial parent's insurance is tertiary (third).

A court order specifying which parent must cover the child's medical expenses supersedes these rules.

When the birthday rule is not followed, some self-funded insurance companies use the gender rule, which states that the father's insurance is always primary.

3. Input Patient Information

Information on the patient information form is then entered into the healthcare facility's medical record and billing system. A medical record and billing system is a computer program used to store and retrieve patient information, bill patients and third-party payers, and track reimbursements.

Although there are different commercial software programs used for this purpose, all of them basically work the same way. There is an initial screen used to enter general information about the patient such as name, address, and Social Security number. There is also a screen to enter information gathered from the medical questionnaire filled out during the patient's first visit. This information includes previous illnesses, allergies, current and previous medications, and other subjective medical information. The program will have a screen used by the healthcare provider to enter the patient's current medical information.

There is also a screen used to enter demographic information from the patient information form. This is where you'll enter the patient's medical insurance information such as the policy number, contacts, type of coverage, restrictions, co-pays, and other data that pertains to billing and reimbursement.

It is very important that information be entered correctly because incorrect information will delay reimbursement. Let's say that the medical insurer will reimburse the full cost of an MRI if the healthcare provider obtains a referral or an authorization for the test from the medical insurer; otherwise there is no reimbursement. If this restriction is noted in the computer, then the healthcare provider will be reminded to ask for approval before scheduling the test. If it isn't, then the healthcare provider may not be reimbursed for the test and in many cases the patient would be held liable for the charges.

Some computer programs will generate the claim and send it electronically to the medical insurer. Once the claim is filed, the computer program is used to track reimbursements.

4. Create an Encounter Form

Creating an encounter form is the next step in the insurance claim cycle. An encounter form (Figure 7–2) is used to record the healthcare provider's encounter with a patient. An encounter might be the patient's visit to the healthcare provider's office or a visit by the healthcare provider to the patient's bedside in the hospital.

The encounter form can be a physical paper form or an electronic form displayed on a computer screen. Sometimes the encounter form is both electronic and paper. In this case, the healthcare provider fills out the paper encounter form, which is then entered into the computer.

The healthcare provider enters on the encounter form the patient's diagnosis and the medical procedure performed on the patient. Each diagnosis and procedure is assigned an ICD-10, CPT-4, and/or HCPCS code. As you learned in Chapter 5, these codes make it easy to communicate a patient's diagnosis and treatment to medical insurers, government health agencies, and other healthcare providers.

Sometimes the encounter form also contains the patient's outstanding balance and a scheduled follow-up appointment. The medical insurance specialist uses the encounter form to post the daily charges prior to submission to the insurance company.

No.	Date	Description	Charge	Credit		Current Balance
				Payment	Adjustment	

Patient Information

Address _____

City, State Zip _____

Home phone _____ Work phone _____

Responsible Person _____
Relationship

Insurance _____ Contract _____
numbers

Patient

_____

Date: _____

Jonathan John, MD

25 S. Edwin Avenue

New York, NY 10023-2240
212-515-7022
Fax: 212-515-0725

Chart # _____

Diagnoses:
1. _____
2. _____
3. _____
4. _____

OFFICE VISITS

New Patient	Established Patient

Preventive Medicine

_____ 99201	_____ 99381 under 1 year	_____ 99391	
	_____ 99382 1–4	_____ 99392	_____ 99211
_____ 99202	_____ 99383 5–11	_____ 99393	_____ 99212
_____ 99203	_____ 99384 12–17	_____ 99394	_____ 99213
_____ 99204	_____ 99385 18–39	_____ 99395	_____ 99214
_____ 99205	_____ 99386 40–64	_____ 99396	_____ 99215
	_____ 99387 65+	_____ 99397	

Hospital Visits

Initial:

_____
99221

_____
99222

_____
99223

Subsequent:

_____
99231

_____
99232

_____
99233

Nursing

Facility

Subsequent:

_____
99311

_____
99312

_____
99313

Other:

_____

_____

Lab:
_____ 80048 Basic metabolic panel (SMA-8)
_____ 87110 Chlamydia culture
_____ 85651 ESR; nonautomated
_____ 83001 FSH
_____ 82947 Glucose, blood
_____ 85022 Hemogram (CBC) with differential
_____ 80076 Hepatic function panel
_____ 85018 HGB
_____ 86701 HIV-1
_____ 83002 LH
_____ 80061 Lipid panel
_____ 86617 Lyme antibody
_____ 86308 Monospot test
_____ 88150 Pap
_____ 85610 Prothrombin time
_____ 84152 PSA

_____ 86430 Rheumatoid factor
_____ 82270 Stool hemoccult x 3
_____ 87430 Strep screen
_____ 84478 Triglycerides
_____ 84443 TSH
_____ 81001 UA with microscopy
_____ 87088 UC
_____ 84550 Uric acid, blood
_____ 81025 Urine pregnancy test
_____
_____
_____
_____

Injections:
_____ 90471 admin 1 vac
_____ 90472 each add'l vac
_____ 90716 Chickenpox
_____ 90702 DT
_____ 90701 DTP
_____ 90657 Influenza 6–35 months
_____ 90658 Influenza 3 years +
_____ 90665 Lyme disease
_____ 90707 MMR
_____ 90704 Mumps
_____ 90713 Polio vac inactivated (IPV)
_____ 90703 Tetanus Tox

ECG: _____ 93000 EKG

Other:
_____
_____
_____

FIGURE 7–2 · Patient encounter form.

The encounter form must be carefully reviewed to make sure that the patient's diagnosis corresponds to the procedure. For example, you wouldn't expect a patient diagnosed with a sore throat to have an X-ray of her foot. Either this was erroneously entered on the form or the patient has another diagnosis that isn't listed on the encounter form.

In addition to examining the encounter form to see if its contents are reasonable, you'll need to also determine if the restrictions set by the medical insurer, such as receiving and documenting referrals from primary-care physicians or preauthorizations, before performing an MRI.

5. Calculate Medical Fees

At this point in the insurance claim cycle, you are ready to calculate medical fees. Typically the healthcare provider has a schedule of fees for each type of encounter whether it is a simple examination or surgery. Sometimes a healthcare provider just writes a dollar amount on the encounter form.

Once fees are totaled for the encounter, you must determine how it will be paid. The patient might decide to pay the entire amount in cash, by check, or by credit card or may have arranged a payment plan with the healthcare provider.

In many cases, the patient's medical insurer will reimburse the healthcare provider for all or part of the fee depending on a number of factors that include the type of medical coverage and the arrangement that the healthcare provider might have with the medical insurer.

A *premium* is the amount of money the insured pays to a medical insurer for a healthcare policy. This fee can be paid monthly, quarterly, semiannually, and annually.

A *deductible* is the amount that the patient will have to pay before the medical insurance will kick in. If a patient has an annual deductible of $500 effective January 1 of every year, the patient must spend down the $500 before the insurance will pay any of the patient's bills. If the patient sees the physician on January 5 and incurs charges of $200, the total amount of the bill will be the patient's responsibility.

The patient's financial responsibilities are not limited to the deductible. Once the deductible has been met, then the medical insurer may only cover a percentage of the cost; for example, the medical insurer may cover 80% of the fee and the patient has to pay the remaining 20%. This division of costs is known as coinsurance.

The medical insurer may cover all but $25, which is the patient's co-payment. This means you collect the payment up front and submit the full charges to the insurance company for processing. The insurer will deduct the patient's co-payment amount from the agreed upon reimbursement fee.

The medical insurer may cover only some of the procedures performed during the encounter, but not all. Therefore, the patient is billed for those not covered and a claim is made for the covered procedures.

The medical insurer may pay a flat fee for the encounter if the healthcare provider has an existing agreement with the medical insurer. You only file a claim for the flat fee, that is, surgical package.

The medical insurer may pay a flat monthly fee to the healthcare provider if he is the patient's primary physician. The monthly fee covers certain types of encounters such as routine office visits. Therefore, there isn't a claim filed with the medical insurer and there isn't a bill presented to the patient. However, the provider may be required to submit an encounter report.

6. Preparing the Claim

With fees totaled, the next step is to create a claims form. There are two methods of claim submissions—paper and electronic. Each requires you to supply the same kinds of information, which is the information that you've gathered from other forms that were filled out during the patient's encounter.

The Insurance Claim section later in this chapter explains in detail how to create a claims form. Before sending the claim to the medical insurer, be sure that the claim form contains clinical and financial information that describes the encounter with the patient. Consult the medical insurer and make sure that you have included all information in the claim form that the medical insurer requires to process the claim. Failure to do this will delay reimbursement.

7. Send the Claim

The claim is sent electronically or by mail to the medical insurer. If you have a choice, always send a claim electronically using software on the healthcare provider's computer because the claim will be received immediately by the medical insurer's computer.

Some benefits of electronic claims are that they

- Decrease processing time.
- Increase reimbursement.

- Secure patient's information.
- Eliminate the risk that the claim will be lost by the post office or other carrier.
- Reduce the paper load because everything is stored in the computer.

8. The Claim Is Received

The claim undergoes the adjudication process when it is received by the medical insurer. During the adjudication process, every aspect of the claim is examined and compared to terms of the group policy that covers the patient.

Claims are not paid unless the medical insurer verifies that

- The patient is covered by the policy.
- The policy covers the encounter.
- The encounter took place (the healthcare provider treated the patient).
- The healthcare provider adhered to any restrictions (i.e., precertifications or approvals).
- The claim is correctly coded.

Once verified, the claim is approved for payment and the healthcare provider is sent a remittance advice (RA) that details all the procedures that were listed on the claim and the reimbursement for each of them. The provider may receive an explanation of benefits (EOBs) from the insurer; however, the EOB is usually sent to the insured. Both the EOB and RA contain the same information. An explanation appears alongside any unreimbursed procedure telling why it wasn't reimbursed. Review the RA carefully, and immediately raise any disputes with the medical insurer.

A medical insurer may postpone sending an RA until it receives more information about a procedure or until the healthcare provider forwards any information that was missing from the claim. The healthcare provider then must provide the additional information; otherwise the provider may not be reimbursed.

And sometimes the RA is sent denying the entire claim. The reason for the denial is specified alongside each procedure on the RA.

The RA is sent by mail or electronically. Reimbursements, if any, are sent by mail or electronically transferred into the healthcare provider's account.

Reimbursements must be recorded on the patient's records immediately when they are received. You should post the reimbursement payments against the charges incurred from each procedure and note any procedures that were denied.

Depending on the healthcare provider, any procedure that was not reimbursed by the healthcare provider can be

- Resubmitted to the medical insurer with appropriate corrections.
- Appealed by submitting documentation that better supports the claim. Every medical insurer has his/her own appeals process; check with the medical insurer or the physician agreement for the regulations.
- Billed to the patient if allowed for the unreimbursed procedure according to the healthcare provider's policy.
- Write off any remaining cost of the procedure as a loss.

9. The Insurance Claim

Now that you know how the insurance claim cycle works, let's take a closer look at the insurance claim itself. Before the medical insurance claim process was streamlined, healthcare providers presented the patient with the bill for the visit and treatment. The patient was expected to pay the healthcare provider before leaving the office and then submit a claim to her medical insurer for reimbursement.

As medical expenses rose, patients were unable to pay the healthcare provider up front and arranged to pay once the reimbursement was received from their medical insurer. Healthcare providers agreed until an unexpected trend developed where some patients did not pay after the reimbursement check had arrived.

Furthermore, the terms and procedures of medical coverage became complex, and medical insurers required medical documentation to support each claim. Patients knew little about medical documentation and found themselves as a go between for the medical insurer and the healthcare provider.

A more efficient system was developed where the patient signed an assignment of benefit consent for payment (located on the Centers for Medicare and Medicaid Services [CMS] 1500 form) that granted the healthcare provider the right to directly file a claim with the patient's medical insurer on the patient's behalf. In doing so, the healthcare provider is responsible to provide the medical insurer with the necessary medical documentation to support the claim—and the medical insurer reimburses the healthcare provider directly. This eliminated the risk that the patient would not pay the healthcare provider.

There are two types of claim forms in use. These are the Health Insurance Portability and Accounting Act (HIPAA) XTT837 form (Figure 7–3), which is an electronic claims format, and the CMS-1500 form (Figure 7–4), which is now only used as a paper claims form. Both formats contain the same type of information.

HIPAA Claim Data Elements

Claim Control Number (Patient Account Number)

PROVIDER, SUBSCRIBER, PATIENT, PAYER

Billing Provider

Last or   City Name
Organization Name   State/Province Code

Middle Name

Name Suffix Primary Identifier: NPI Address 1 Address 2 City Name State/Province Code ZIP Code
Country Code

Secondary Identifiers, such as State License Number Contact Name Communication Numbers

Telephone Number
Fax
E-mail
Telephone Extension Taxonomy Code Currency Code

Pay-to Provider

Last or Organization Name

First Name
Middle Name
Name Suffix Primary Identifier: NPI Address 1 Address 2 City Name State/Province Code

ZIP Code

Country Code

Secondary Identifiers, such as State License Number

Taxonomy Code

Subscriber

Insured Group or Policy Number
Group or Plan Name
Insurance Type Code
Claim Filing Indicator Code
Last Name
First Name
Middle Name
Name Suffix
Primary Identifier Member Identification Number National Individual Identifier IHS/CHS Tribe
Residency Code

FIGURE 7–3 • HIPAA XTT837 claims form.

Secondary Identifiers HIS Health Record Number Insurance Policy Number SSN

Patient's Relationship to Subscriber
Other Subscriber Information
 Birth Date
Gender Code
Address Line 1
Address Line 2

Country Code
Patient
Last Name First Name Middle Name Name Suffix Primary Identifier
    Member ID Number

National Individual identifier Address 1

Address 2

City Name State/Province Code

Zip Code

Country Code

Birth Date

Gender Code

Secondary Identifiers

    IHS Health Record Number
    Insurance Policy Number
    SSN
Death Date

Weight

Pregnancy Indicator

Responsible Party

Last or Organization Name
First Name
Middle Name
Suffix Name
Address 1
Address 2
City Name
State/Province Code
Zip Code
Country Code

Payer

Payer Responsibility Sequence Number Code

 Organization Name

Primary Identifier

    Payer ID

    National Plan ID

Address 1

 Address 2

City Name

 State/Province Code

Zip Code

Secondary Identifiers

    Claim Office Number

    NAIC Code

    TIN

Assignment of Benefits

 Release of Information Code

Patient Signature Source Code

 Referral Number

Prior Authorization Number

FIGURE 7–3 · (*Continued*)

HIPAA Claim Data Elements *(Continued)*

Claim Control Number (Patient Account Number)

Claim Level

Total Submitted Charges
Place of Service Code
Claim Frequency Code
Provider Signature on File
Medicare Assignment Code
Participation Agreement
Delay Reason Code
Onset of Current Symptoms or illness Date
Similar Illness/Symptom Onset Date
Claim Original Reference Number
Investigational Device Exemption Last
    Menstrual Period Date
Admission Date
Discharge Date
Patient Amount Paid

Number

Medical Record Number
Note Reference Code
Claim Note
Diagnosis Code 1–8
Accident Claims

> Accident Cause Auto Accident
> Another Party Responsible
> Employment Related Other
> Accident
>
> Auto Accident State/Province
>   Code
> Auto Accident Country Code
> Accident Date
> Accident Hour

Rendering Provider _____

Last or Organization Name

First Name

Middle Name Name Suffix
Primary Identifier
    EIN
    NPI
    SSN
Taxonomy Code Secondary
Identifiers

Referring/PCP Providers
Last or Organization Name First
Name Middle Name Name Suffix
Primary Identifier
    EIN
    NPI
    SSN
Taxonomy Code Secondary
Identifiers Proc Service Facility
Location
Type Code
Last or Organization Name
Primary Identifier
    EIN
    NPI
    SSN
Address 1 Address 2 City Name
State/Province Code Zip Code
Country Code Secondary
Identifiers

SERVICE LINE INFORMATION

Procedure Type Code
Procedure Code
Modifiers 1–4
Line Item Charge Amount
Units of Service/Anesthesia
Minutes
Place of Service Code
Diagnosis Code Pointers 1–4
Emergency Indicator
Copay Status Code
Service Date Begun
Service Date End

Shipped Date
Onset Date
Similar Illness or Symptom Date
Referral/Prior Authorization Number
Line Item Control Number
Ambulatory Patient Group
Sales Tax Amount
Postage Claimed Amount
Line Note Text
Rendering/Referring/PCP Provider at the Service
    Line Level
Service Facility Location at the Service Line Level

FIGURE 7–3 · *(Continued)*

PLEASE
DO NOT
STAPLE
IN THIS
AREA

CARRIER

HEALTH INSURANCE CLAIM FORM

☐☐☐PICA   PICA ☐☐☐

1. MEDICARE   MEDICAD   CHAMPUS   CHAMPVA   GROUP   FECA   OTHER   1a. INSURED'S I.D. NUMBER   (FOR PROGRAM IN ITEM 1)
                                                HEALTH PLAN BLKLUNG
☐ (Medicare #) ☐ (Medicaid #) ☐ (Sponsor's SSN) ☐ (VA File #) ☐ (SSN or ID) ☐ (SSN) ☐ (ID)

2. PATIENT'S NAME (Last Name, First Name, Middle Initial)   3. PATIENT'S BIRTH DATE   SEX   4. INSURED'S NAME (Last Name, First Name, Middle Initial)
                                                            MM   DD   YY
                                                                            M ☐   F ☐

5. PATIENT'S ADDRESS (NO., Street)   6. PATIENT RELATIONSHIP TO INSURED   7. INSURED'S ADDRESS (NO., Street)
                                                            Self ☐ Spouse ☐ Child ☐ Other ☐

CITY   STATE   8. PATIENT STATUS   CITY   STATE
                                                            Single ☐ Married ☐ Other ☐

ZIP CODE   TELEPHONE (Include Area Code)   ZIP CODE   TELEPHONE (INCLUDE AREA CODE)
                       (   )   Employed ☐ Full-Time ☐ Part-Time ☐   (   )
                                                                        Student   Student

9. OTHER INSURED'S NAME (Last Name, First Name, Middle Initial)   10. IS PATIENT'S CONDITION RELATED TO: 11. INSURED'S POLICY GROUP OR FECA NUMBER

a. OTHER INSURED'S POLICY OR GROUP NUMBER   a. EMPLOYMENT? (CURRENT OR PREVIOUS)   a. INSURED'S DATE OF BIRTH   SEX
                                                                    ☐ YES   ☐ NO   MM   DD   YY   M ☐   F ☐

b. OTHER INSURED'S DATE OF BIRTH   SEX   b. AUTO ACCIDENT?   PLACE (State)   b. EMPLOYER'S NAME OR SCHOOL NAME
   MM   DD   YY   M ☐   F ☐   ☐ YES   ☐ NO

c. EMPLOYER'S NAME OR SCHOOL NAME   c. OTHER ACCIDENT?   c. INSURANCE PLAN NAME OR PROGRAM NAME
                                                                    ☐ YES   ☐ NO

d. INSURANCE PLAN NAME OR PROGRAM NAME   10d. RESERVED FOR LOCAL USE   d. IS THERE ANOTHER HEALTH BENEFIT PLAN?
                                                                                                   ☐ YES   ☐ NO   If yes, return to and complete item 9 a-d.

READ BACK OF FORM BEFORE COMPLETING & SIGNING THIS FORM.
12. PATIENT'S OR AUTHORIZED PERSON'S SIGNATURE I authorize the release of any medical or other information necessary   13. INSURED'S OR AUTHORIZED PERSON'S SIGNATURE I authorize
to process this claim. I also request payment of government benefits either to myself or to the party who accepts assignment   payment of medical benefits to the undersigned physician or supplier
below.   for services described below.

SIGNED _____   DATE _____   SIGNED _____

14. DATE OF CURRENT: ☐ ILLNESS (First symptom) OR   15. IF PATIENT HAS HAD SAME OR SIMILAR ILLNESS.   16. DATES PATIENT UNABLE TO WORK IN CURRENT OCCUPATION
   MM   DD   YY   INJURY (Accident) OR   GIVE FIRST DATE   MM   DD   YY   MM   DD   YY   MM   DD   YY
                       PREGNANCY (LMP)   FROM   TO

17. NAME OF REFERRING PHYSICIAN OR OTHER SOURCE   17a. I.D. NUMBER OF REFERRING PHYSICIAN   18. HOSPITALIZATION DATES RELATED TO CURRENT SERVICES
                                                                                                   MM   DD   YY   MM   DD   YY
                                                                                                 FROM   TO

19. RESERVED FOR LOCAL USE   20. OUTSIDE LAB? $ CHARGES
                                                                                                   ☐ YES   ☐ NO

21. DIAGNOSIS OR NATURE OF ILLNESS OR INJURY. (RELATE ITEMS 1, 2, 3 OR 4 TO ITEM 24E BY LINE)   22. MEDICAID RESUBMISSION
                                                                                                   CODE   ORIGINAL REF. NO.
1. ⌊___.___   3. ⌊___.___
                                                                                                  23. PRIOR AUTHORIZATION NUMBER
2. ⌊___.___   4. ⌊___.___

24. A		B	C	D	E	F	G	H	I	J	K
DATE(S) OF SERVICE		Place	Type	PROCEDURES, SERVICES, OR SUPPLIES	DIAGNOSIS		DAYS	EPSDT			RESERVED FOR
From	To	of	of	(Explain Unusual Circumstances)	CODE	$ CHARGES	OR	Family	EMG	COB	LOCAL USE
MM DD YY	MM DD YY	Service	Service	CPT/HCPCS MODIFIER			UNITS	Plan			

25. FEDERAL TAX I.D. NUMBER   SSN EIN   26. PATIENT'S ACCOUNT NO.   27. ACCEPT ASSIGNMENT?   28. TOTAL CHARGE   29. AMOUNT PAID   30. BALANCE DUE
                               ☐ ☐   (For govt. claims, see back) $ $ $
                                                                     ☐ YES   ☐ NO

31. SIGNATURE OF PHYSICIAN OR SUPPLIER   32. NAME AND ADDRESS OF FACILITY WHERE SERVICES WERE   33. PHYSICIAN'S, SUPPLIER'S BILLING NAME, ADDRESS, ZIP CODE
INCLUDING DEGREES OR CREDENTIALS   RENDERED (If other than home or office)   & PHONE #
(I certify that the statements on the reverse
apply to this bill and are made a part the reof.)

SIGNED _____   DATE _____   PIN#   GRP#

(APPROVED BY AMA COUNCIL ON MEDICAL SERVICE 8/89)   PLEASE PRINT OR TYPE   APPROVED OMB-0938-0008 FORM CMS-1500 (12/00), FORM RRB-1500,
                                                                             APPROVED OMB-1215-0055 FORM OWCP-1500, APPROVED CMB-0720-0001 (CHAMPUS)

PATIENT AND INSURED INFORMATION

PHYSICIAN OR SUPPLIER INFORMATION

FIGURE 7–4 · CMS-1500 claims form.

In the claim you must answer the following questions:

- Is the patient's condition related to employment, an auto accident, or another kind of accident?
- Does the patient have additional insurance coverage?
- Were the services of an outside laboratory used in the diagnosis of the patient?
- Does the healthcare provider accept assignment (reimbursement allowed by the medical insurer)?

Nearly all the information required for a claim is available from the medical billing computer software that is used by the healthcare provider.

10. HIPAA Claims and Paper Claims

Congress passed the HIPAA in 1996. This law was developed and implemented by the Centers for Medicare and Medicaid Services. One of the provisions in the law pertains to the creation of a standardized electronic claims format, the XTT837.

The HIPAA XTT837 claims format, commonly referred to as an *837 claim*, is transmitted electronically to the medical insurer. Before the 837 claim was mandated by the HIPAA law, healthcare providers submitted a CMS-1500 paper or electronic claims form to medical insurers. This claims form was usually printed by a medical billing computer software and then mailed, faxed, or submitted electronically to the medical insurer for processing. The CMS requested that an electronic version of the CMS-1500 claims form be used for submitting Medicare claims.

During the era of paper medical insurance claims forms, each medical insurer had his/her own diagnoses and procedural coding system. However, this changed when HIPAA law required that the ICD-10-CM, CPT, and HCPCS codes were to be used as the standard code sets. The HIPAA law also mandated the use of the new electronic claims format created by the CMS.

HIPAA Data Elements

The HIPAA 837 claims form (see Figure 7–3) is divided into five major sections referred to as *levels.* These are

1. Provider
2. Subscriber (guarantor, insured, policyholder) and patient
3. Insurance company

4. Claim details

5. Services

These levels form a hierarchy of information that minimizes the need to duplicate information among levels. The first level describes the provider. The second level profiles the subscriber and the patient. The subscriber is the person who is issued the medical insurance. The patient may or may not also be the subscriber. For example, a child might be the patient and his parent the subscriber.

Some information is required depending on the nature of the encounter. For example, the medical insurer only needs to know the patient's last menstrual period if pregnancy is diagnosed.

You might be unfamiliar with some terms used in each level. These are described in Table 7–1.

CMS-1500 Data Elements

The CMS-1500 claims form (see Figure 7–4) is organized into 34 form locators. A form locator is an area where you enter information onto the form. Each form locator is identified by a unique number.

TABLE 7–1 Terms Contained in Each Level of the Hipaa 873 Claims Form

Term	Description
Referral/prior authorization number	A number issued by a medical insurer when preapproval is given to a healthcare provider to perform a procedure on the patient
Line item control number	Number assigned to each line of service on an electronic claim. Used to track payments from the insurance carrier for a particular service rather than the entire claim
Billing provider	The provider submitting the bill (e.g., the billing service)
Type/place of service codes	Type of service patient received (e.g., medical, emergency). Place of service where the services occurred
Taxonomy code	A 10-digit code that stands for a physician's medical specialty
Line note text	This is where the healthcare provider can insert a comment
Rendering/referring/PCP provider at the service line level	Name of the physician who provided the service
Service facility location at the service line level	Address of the site where services were provided

Similar to the HIPAA 873 claims form, form locators on the CMS-1500 claims form are organized into two main groups. These are patient information (locators 1 through 13) and healthcare provider and transactional information (locators 14 through 34).

11. Health Insurance Portability and Accounting Act

As previously stated, in 1996, Congress instituted the HIPAA to provide a way for a person to continue healthcare coverage while between employers. However, Congress expanded this act in 2003 to protect patient privacy and standardize electronic claims transmission and processing.

Patients have the right to determine how their personal and medical information is used for treatment, payment of medical bills, and within a healthcare facility. Patient information is shared on a need-to-know basis as required to perform a specific task. For example, a medical insurance specialist needs to know what laboratory tests were performed and the fees for those tests, but not the test results.

Besides ensuring patient privacy, HIPAA defined the format used to store patient medical information electronically. This is referred to as the *HIPAA transaction set*. Think of this as defining the way all medical insurers and healthcare providers must electronically store and transmit claims. However, this standard does not apply to claims transmitted on paper through the mail, by fax, or conveyed over the telephone.

All healthcare providers who have more than 10 employees are required to use the HIPAA transaction set when filing Medicare claims.

12. Types of Health Insurance Coverage

Filing a claim is complicated because there are many types of medical coverage that are available to patients. Each is designed to provide the best, cost-effective care to meet the medical needs of different kinds of patients.

Health insurance coverage falls into one of three categories: traditional coverage, managed care, and government.

Traditional Coverage

Traditional coverage is a fee-for-service plan where a medical insurer pays 80% of medical costs and the patient pays the remaining 20% of the fee. There are restrictions that apply in traditional coverage. For example, a waiting period might be imposed before the policy takes effect during which time the patient is not reimbursed for medical expenses.

In traditional coverage

- The patient does not need to select a primary physician who would coordinate the patient's medical care. Referrals to medical specialists are not necessary. Patients are free to seek care from whichever provider they choose.

- A coordination of benefits statement is used to specify that medical expenses will be shared between insurers if the patient is covered by two or more medical policies as in the case where a child is covered under each parent's medical plan.

- Reimbursement can be made directly to the patient for medical expenses.

Basic Insurance

Basic medical insurance is a traditional coverage that has a maximum reimbursement amount written into the policy. The patient pays all medical expenses that exceed the maximum set in the policy.

Reimbursement is based on either usual and customary fees or a specified amount for each procedure. A usual and customary fee is the fee that physicians within the geographic area charge most patients for a service. Let's say that a physician charges $1,000 for a procedure and the medical insurer determines the usual and customary fee for that procedure is $750; then the patient pays $250.

Many basic policies have a deductible or co-payment such as $100 deductible or $25 co-payment. If a visit to a physician costs $200 and the policy has a $100 deductible, the patient is responsible to pay the $100 and the balance is paid to the healthcare provider by the medical insurer. If the policy has a $25 co-payment, the patient must pay $25 and the medical insurer pays the rest of the medical expenses to the healthcare provider.

Some basic policies have annual deductibles. For example, suppose the policy has a $1,000 annual deductible for hospital care. The patient visits the emergency room twice incurring a $500 charge each time. The patient won't receive any reimbursement from the insurer because the patient is required to pay the first $1,000.

A patient who has basic medical coverage may find restrictions on hospital care. For example, the policy may reimburse for a specific number of days in the hospital or limit reimbursement to a semiprivate room. The patient must pay for anything not covered by the policy.

Major Medical Insurance

Major medical insurance is also a traditional coverage that reimburses for medical catastrophes that require extensive and expensive treatment. Typically, major medical coverage has a 20% deductible provision referred to as *coinsurance* that is paid for by the patient.

The major medical coverage usually reimburses the insured the percentage specified in the policy, that is, 80% of total amount paid. It also covers services that are not normally covered in basic coverage. These include medical equipment rental or purchase, special nursing care, and prosthetic devices.

Comprehensive major medical insurance is an extended major medical policy that provides coverage similar to basic coverage and major medical coverage. Nearly all medical conditions are covered under this policy.

Blue Cross and Blue Shield

As you'll recall from Chapter 1, Blue Cross and Blue Shield is a not-for-profit organization that provides traditional medical coverage for a fixed premium regardless of how often a patient receives medical care.

Blue Shield is an insurance that reimburses patients for healthcare provider services such as a visit to a physician's office. Blue Cross reimburses for hospital care. A patient can subscribe to one or both plans.

Besides traditional coverage, Blue Cross and Blue Shield has expanded its offerings to include managed-care plans.

Managed-Care Models

Managed care is a category different from traditional coverage. It is designed to keep patients healthy by giving them preventive care. Managed care is an evolving area of healthcare that has a different structure from traditional coverage. In some managed-care plans, a patient's medical expenses are completely covered if the patient uses a preferred healthcare provider.

The more common managed-care plans are health maintenance organizations (HMOs), exclusive provider organizations (EPO), preferred provider organizations (PPO), Integrated Delivery System (IDS), the point-of-service (POS) plan, and the triple option plan.

Health Maintenance Organizations

An HMO offers healthcare provider services and hospital care at little or no cost to the patient except for either a monthly or annual payment. Each patient selects a primary physician who is paid a fixed monthly fee for each patient regardless of the care the patient is given. This physician has a financial incentive to provide preventive care. A patient who avoids illness frees up the physician to see other patients, while still receiving the monthly fee for the healthy patient.

Some HMOs operate clinics staffed by salaried physicians. Patients can use these services at any time at no charge. Other HMOs contract with a group of physicians who collectively care for HMO patients.

The medical expenses for patients are fully covered if they use HMO-owned or HMO-contracted physicians and healthcare facilities. HMOs usually cover emergency care given by any healthcare provider.

Some HMOs require patients to pay a co-payment from $5 to $25 each time the patient uses the HMO's facilities. This includes prescription medication.

HMOs have a financial incentive to provide patients with care that prevents illness so they avoid expensive emergency and hospital care. Furthermore, HMOs reduce the need for unnecessary and duplicate laboratory procedures. It also removes the incentive for some healthcare providers to perform unnecessary procedures in order to increase their reimbursement.

Some patients don't use HMOs for fear that healthcare providers will forgo medical tests in order to reduce expenses.

Exclusive Provider Organization

EPO is another type of managed-care plan coverage. Patients must use only healthcare providers and facilities that are in the EPO's network. The patient can use services outside the network but won't be reimbursed for those expenses.

An EPO contracts with healthcare providers and healthcare facilities to provide services for a fixed rate. Patients are charged a fixed monthly rate for coverage.

Preferred Provider Organization

A PPO provides medical coverage to a group such as union members or employees of a company. The group must agree to use physicians and healthcare facilities that are associated with the PPO.

The PPO negotiates low healthcare fees by promising to refer large numbers of patients to associated physicians and healthcare facilities. The PPO doesn't own healthcare facilities nor does it have physicians on staff. Instead associates operate on a traditional fee-for-service arrangement except fees are lower for PPO patients than for non-PPO patients. Patients are fully covered and pay a co-payment and a premium to the PPO.

Integrated Delivery System

An IDS is a managed-care plan where groups of physicians and ambulatory centers join together to offer patients medical care in exchange for a fixed monthly fee. Patients can choose their physician from among those who are in the IDS. Models include physician–hospital organizations, management services organizations, group practices without walls, integrated provider organizations, and medical foundations.

Point-of-Service Plan

A POS plan gives patients the option of going to a physician or medical facility that is in the POS network or to any healthcare provider that is outside the network. The POS typically requires a patient to pay a very high deductible or co-payment when they go out-of-network for healthcare. The deductible can be as high as several hundred dollars and the co-payment nearly a quarter of the healthcare provider's fee.

Triple Option Plan

The triple option plan (also known as the *cafeteria plan*) gives patients a choice of traditional coverage, HMO, or preferred provider service. This type of plan is usually offered by one or more insurers; it provides employees with a choice of plans as well as insurance carriers. Triple option plans are intended to prevent the problem of covering members who are sicker than the general population—called *adverse selection*. A risk pool is created when a number of people are grouped for insurance purposes (eg, employees of an organization); the cost of healthcare coverage is determined by an employee's health status, age, sex, and occupation.

Health Savings Account Plan

Health saving account plans enable the insured to place pre-tax dollars into an account. The insured can then use funds in the account to pay out-of-pocket expenses for medical care that is covered by the insured's health insurance policy. Only services covered by the health insurance policy can be paid for by funds from the health savings account plan.

Government Insurance Plans

Federal and state governments provide one of the largest kinds of medical coverage. As the baby boomers reach retirement age, they will be turning to government programs to provide medical care.

As you learned in Chapter 1, Medicare and Medicaid are the primary government medical programs that care for medical expenses for the elderly and the poor. There are also other government programs that cover the federal employees and workers who get injured on the job.

Medicare

Medicare is the federal government medical insurance program that covers Americans who are 65 years and older and Americans who have disabilities. Medicare coverage is divided into four categories referred to as *Part A, B, C,* and *D*. Part A reimburses for hospital expenses and Part B covers nonhospital expenses such as visits to healthcare providers.

Part A covers most—but not all—of the expenses that are related to a patient's hospital care. Part B covers 80% of a healthcare provider's reasonable fee for treating the patient. The patient is expected to pay the remaining 20% of the fee.

Medicare is administered by the CMS. However, the CMS contracts with large insurance companies to process Medicare claims for each state.

It is important that you contact your local Medicare office for the name of the firm who processes Medicare claims for your state. Contact that firm and ask it to explain its claims processing to you. Each firm that processes Medicare claims has a slightly different claims procedure. If you do not know those procedures, reimbursement may be delayed. Sometimes different firms process Part A and Part B claims.

A Medicare patient may be covered by one or both parts. Ask Medicare patients for their Medicare card. It will show their coverage plus their Medicare identification number, which you will need to file a Medicare claim.

When a healthcare provider accepts a Medicare patient, it also accepts Medicare's scheduled reimbursement as 80% payment for its services. The patient pays 20%. Fees that exceed these amounts cannot be charged to the patient. Instead, the healthcare provider writes them off as a loss.

Premiums for Part A coverage are indirectly paid for by payroll taxes.

Part B covers outpatient services. Premiums are deducted monthly from the patient's Social Security check.

Part C, commonly called *Medicare Advantage Plans* or MA Plans, is coverage offered by private companies that are approved by Medicare. Part C offers hospital insurance (Medicare Part A) and medical insurance (Medicare Part B). These are the same Medicare services covered by Medicare; however, the MA Plans—not Medicare—pay for services. MA Plans may offer extra coverage that is not covered under Medicare. MA Plans may have different rules on how the insured receives care such as limited services to selected providers and requiring referrals to a specialist. Likewise, MA Plans can charge different out-of-pocket cost.

Part D, commonly called *Medicare Prescription Drug Plan*, covers prescription medication coverage to Medicare, Medicare Medical Savings Account (MSA) plans, Medicare Cost Plans, and Medicare Private Fee-for-Service Plans. Drug coverage is also covered through MA Plans, commonly referred to as *MA-PDs*.

Medicaid

Medicaid is a joint federal and state program that provides medical coverage to the poor. Medicaid can reimburse the 20% of medical expenses that Medicare doesn't pay for individuals who qualify of medical expenses that Medicare doesn't pay. Medicaid coverage and claim procedures are determined by each state. Therefore, you'll need to contact your local Medicaid office to determine coverage and claim procedures for your state.

It is important to understand that states impose a time limit for filing Medicaid claims; the time limit differs from state to state. The Medicaid claim will be rejected if the claim is filed beyond this deadline.

Make sure that you ask for the patient's Medicaid identification card. This card contains information that you will need to file a claim.

Workers' Compensation Insurance

Workers' compensation insurance is medical coverage that states require employers to purchase for their employees and that provides healthcare coverage and income protection to an employee and dependents if the employee suffers or dies from a work-related injury or illness.

Although the law requires the employer to purchase workers' compensation insurance, private insurance companies offer this coverage. Employers pay the entire premium for this coverage. Some states exclude domestic workers, farmers, and small companies from this law.

The patient's medical expenses are covered from the time of the injury or diagnosis of the illness until the patient completely recovers. A worker who is disabled receives income benefits. Dependents receive moderate funeral expenses and living expenses if the worker dies as a result of a work-related injury or illness.

Contact your state's Bureau of Workers' Compensation to learn about coverage and claim processing for workers' compensation insurance. Each state has different coverage and processing requirements. You'll also need to contact the patient's employer for documentation of the patient's injury or illness.

Other Government Programs

Federal government employees, such as military personnel, receive medical coverage under a special insurance program. Many medical insurance specialists won't submit claims to these programs unless their healthcare provider is affiliated with one of these programs. Your healthcare provider can help you contact the administrator of these programs to learn their claim procedures.

These programs include

- **Civilian Health and Medical Program of the Uniformed Services (CHAMPUS).** Covers medical care for military service personnel and their dependents for medical conditions that are not related to military service. Most patients covered by CHAMPUS receive medical care from government healthcare facilities. However, they can receive treatment from nongovernment healthcare providers and healthcare facilities by referral from a government healthcare provider or by choice. In these situations, the commander of the patient's military hospital must authorize the treatment by issuing the private healthcare provider a statement of authorization. This statement must be submitted with the medical claim to CHAMPUS for reimbursement.

- **Civilian Health and Medical Program of the Veterans Administration (CHAMPVA).** Provides coverage for dependents of totally disabled veterans whose disabilities are service related and for surviving dependents of veterans who have died from service-related disabilities.

- **Federal Employees' Health Benefits Program (FEHB).** Covers active and retired federal employees and their dependents. FEHB is administered by the Civil Service Commission which contracts with private insurers to provide coverage.

- **TRICARE.** A managed-care plan for employees, retirees, and their dependents of the Public Health Service and the North Atlantic Treaty Organization (NATO). TRICARE cares for nonmilitary service-related conditions and offers three types of coverage: standard basic fee-for-service, extra preferred provider, and prime where healthcare is managed by a primary healthcare provider in a military treatment facility.

CASE STUDY

CASE 1
You apply for a medical coding and billing position and have been called in for an interview. One of the principal practitioners for the medical group asks you the following questions about the insurance claim cycle. What is your best response?

QUESTION 1. What is the insurance claim cycle?
ANSWER: The insurance claim cycle is a process that you follow to bill a third-party payer for a patient's medical care and to receive appropriate and timely payment.

QUESTION 2. Why is a patient asked to sign an assignment of benefit and release form?
ANSWER: By signing this form, the patient permits the healthcare provider to file a claim directly with the patient's medical insurer and allows the medical insurer to reimburse the healthcare provider. Furthermore, it also authorizes the healthcare provider to share the patient's medical information with the medical insurer.

QUESTION 3. What is the verification of insurance process?
ANSWER: You must immediately verify that the policy is active, whether the patient requires a referral, the type of plan, and the deductible information if any to ensure the healthcare provider will be reimbursed for the patient's medical cost. Although the patient's medical insurance card identifies that the patient has medical coverage, it is insufficient verification because the policy might have lapsed.

QUESTION 4. If a child's parents are divorced, whose healthcare policy covers the child?
ANSWER: If the patient is a child of divorced parents and is covered by policies provided by both parents' employers, then the custodial parent's insurance is primary. If the parent remarries, then the custodial stepparent's plan becomes secondary and the noncustodial parent's insurance becomes tertiary (third). A court order specifying which parent must cover the child's medical expenses supersedes these rules. When the birthday rule is not followed, some self-funded insurance companies use the gender rule, which states that the father's insurance is always primary.

FINAL CHECKUP

1. **How can you verify that a patient's health insurance is active?**
   A. Ask the patient.
   B. Ask the patient to show the health insurance ID card.
   C. Use the medical insurer's Web site, by telephone, or through an insurance eligibility verification system.
   D. Ask the practitioner.

2. **If the patient has two jobs and each employer provides health insurance, which policy is the primary policy?**
   A. The policy that is in effect the longest is the primary policy.
   B. The policy that is in effect the shortest is the primary policy.
   C. Either policy can be considered the primary policy.
   D. The patient selects which of the policies is the primary policy.

3. **What is a healthcare encounter?**
   A. An encounter is whenever the patient calls the practitioner's office.
   B. An encounter is whenever the patient engages the practitioner for service.
   C. An encounter is whenever the patient pays a co-pay.
   D. An encounter is whenever the patient's insurer pays a reimbursement.

4. **A deductible is the amount that the patient will have to pay before the medical insurance will pay a reimbursement.**
   A. True
   B. False

5. **During the adjudication process, every aspect of the claim is examined and compared to terms of the group policy that covers the patient.**
   A. True
   B. False

6. **What happens when a claim is approved by the insurer?**
   A. Once the claim is approved for payment, and the medical billing and coding professional sends the insurer a remittance advice (RA) that details all the procedures that were listed on the claim and the reimbursement for each of them.
   B. Once the claim is approved for payment, the patient sends the insurer an RA that details all the procedures that were listed on the claim and the reimbursement for each of them.
   C. Once the claim is approved for payment, the healthcare provider sends an RA that details all the procedures that were listed on the claim and the reimbursement for each of them.

D. Once verified, the claim is approved for payment and the healthcare provider is sent an RA that details all the procedures that were listed on the claim and the reimbursement for each of them.

7. **Emdeon or Passport are systems used to assist patient pay co-payments.**

   A. True
   B. False

8. **What is the easiest way to gather a patient's health insurance information?**

   A. Ask the patient to tell you the information.
   B. Ask the patient to complete an insurance information form.
   C. Make a copy of the patient's health insurance card.
   D. Call the patient's health insurer.

9. **If the patient is a child who lives with both parents and is covered by two medical policies—provided by each parent's employer—primary coverage is provided by the employer of the parent whose birthday comes second in the calendar year.**

   A. True
   B. False

10. **Patient information entered incorrectly into the healthcare facility's records can delay reimbursements.**

    A. True
    B. False

CORRECT ANSWERS AND RATIONALES

1. **C.** Use the medical insurer's Web site, by telephone, or through an insurance eligibility verification system.
2. **A.** The policy that is in effect the longest is the primary policy.
3. **B.** An encounter is whenever the patient engages the practitioner for service.
4. **A.** True.
5. **A.** True.
6. **D.** Once verified, the claim is approved for payment and the healthcare provider is sent a remittance advice (RA) that details all the procedures that were listed on the claim and the reimbursement for each of them.
7. **B.** False.
8. **C.** Make a copy of the patient's health insurance card.
9. **B.** False.
10. **A.** True.

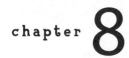

chapter **8**

Billing and Coding Errors: How to Avoid Them

LEARNING OBJECTIVES

1. The Hidden Cost of Errors
2. Types of Errors
3. Dumb Mistakes
4. Red Flags
5. The Penalty for Coding Errors

KEY TERMS

Assumption Coding

Identification on Support Documents

Improper Documentation

Intact Claim Form

Mismatch Coding

Noncompliance

Omissions

Preapproval

Reconstructing Documentation

Truncated Coding

Typographical Errors

Unbundling

Up Coding/Down Coding

1. The Hidden Cost of Errors

A constant, dependable stream of reimbursements from insurers is the blood that keeps a medical practice and a healthcare facility alive. Any disruption of that stream has nearly the same effect as a patient who is bleeding. As the stream slows, the medical practice or healthcare facility slowly dies.

Reimbursements stop flowing when insurers deny claims or delay processing them. And coding and billing errors are the major reasons why this happens. Honest—and sometimes dumb—mistakes cause insurers to withhold reimbursements until the healthcare provider submits a correct claim.

The medical insurance specialist's responsibility is to keep reimbursements flowing by making sure all claims are error-free before a claim is sent to an insurer for processing.

Billing and coding errors can have far-reaching effects because errors disrupt cash flowing into the operation—cash is needed to pay expenses including salaries. Healthcare facilities and medical practices both incur weekly and monthly expenses before they receive money from third-party payers or directly from patients.

Mortgage, rent, utility bills, equipment purchases, and employees' compensation are some of the expenses that must be paid before the first patient walks through the door. Reimbursements are the primary revenue source although a relatively small amount is received as either co-payments or fully paid fees by patients.

Reimbursement occurs only if claims are submitted shortly after care is delivered to the patient and if third-party payers approve those claims. Any delay might cause the practice or healthcare facility to seek temporary revenue sources, such as bank loans called *revolving credit,* until claims are reimbursed. This is very similar to a credit card where arrangements are made in advance for a line of credit. Money can be borrowed as needed without having to apply for a bank loan each time. And just like credit cards, banks charge interest on funds borrowed from a revolving credit account, which is another expense that must be paid using the reimbursement.

Many medical practices and healthcare facilities develop an ongoing flow of cash where reimbursements from previously submitted claims arrive in time to cover expenses incurred delivering healthcare services to current patients. However, this flow of cash can easily be disrupted if claims are not properly prepared and submitted. Therefore, it is critical that the medical insurance specialist carefully examines each claim for common errors before submitting them for processing by third-party payers.

Patient relations are also negatively impacted when a claim is denied. Although a patient signs an acknowledgment that she will pay for fees not covered by her insurer, many patients don't expect to pay anything except possibly a co-pay.

The insurer notifies the patient when a claim is denied leading the patient to believe she is responsible for additional, and possibly substantial, medical expenses. For most patients, healthcare and medical insurance claims are foreign to them. Their insurer and healthcare provider take care of all the medical and insurance details. The notice sent by the insurer is alarming. Besides being exposed to unexpected medical expenses, it also implies that the patient received unnecessary treatment by the healthcare provider.

Besides affecting cash flow and patient relations, medical billing and coding errors can lead to an investigation by regulators or law enforcement agencies. An innocent mistake might be taken as evidence of possible fraud. It is the job of investigators to examine the records of the practice or healthcare facility to determine if this is an inadvertent mistake or something more sinister.

During the course of the investigation, investigators examine the claim in question and other claims to decide if there is a pattern of fraud. Even if there isn't fraud, investigators might uncover discrepancies that cause settled claims to be denied.

Furthermore, the practice or healthcare facility incurs unexpected expenses, such as attorney's fees, during an investigation. The medical insurance specialist and other staff members are diverted from filing new claims as they provide investigators with documentation.

2. Types of Errors

Not all errors can be eliminated; however, by recognizing the more common ones you can take steps to avoid them—and in doing so ensure that the cash flow to the medical practice or healthcare facility isn't unnecessarily disrupted.

Let's take a look at the more common claims errors that medical insurance specialists can make even after being on the job for years.

- **Assumption coding.** This happens when the medical insurance specialist assumes that the healthcare provider administered standard treatment to a patient who is diagnosed with a routine illness when in fact the health-care provider didn't. This error is easily picked up by the third-party pay-er's claims processing system, which automatically withholds reimbursement until the healthcare provider supplies supporting documents.

- **Truncated coding.** This occurs when claims contain a diagnosis code that isn't at its highest level of specificity. As you'll recall from Chapter 6, there are three levels of diagnosis codes: manifestation, episode of care, and site of infliction. A truncated code contains the first or maybe the second level but not all three levels.

- **Mismatch coding.** This occurs when an element of the claim is not con-sistent with other elements, such as the gender is coded as male for a diagnosis of a hysterectomy.

- **Improper documentation.** This is documentation submitted with the claim that is inaccurate or incomplete. The claim is either rejected or reimbursements are withheld until proper documentation is submitted to the third-party payer.

- **Reconstructing documentation.** This happens when supporting docu-mentation is re-created or existing documentation is altered to support a claim submitted to a third-party payer. Altering documents exposes the healthcare provider to civil and criminal charges of fraud.

- **Noncompliance.** Claims must adhere to policies of a third-party payer; otherwise reimbursement will be denied. Let's say that two physicians from the same medical practice examine the same patient on the same day in the hospital—one in the morning and the other in the afternoon. Only one of them will be reimbursed for the examination. The claim will be rejected if both seek reimbursement.

- **Preapproval.** Third-party payers require preapproval before the health-care provider performs certain medical procedures. The claim will be denied if the procedure is performed without the approval of the third-party payer. The healthcare provider can perform the procedure before seeking approval, but he is taking a gamble that the third-party payer will ultimately approve the procedure.

- **Up coding/down coding.** Up coding occurs when the claim contains a procedure code that is reimbursed at a higher rate than the procedure actually performed on the patient. Up coding exposes the healthcare provider to an investigation and risk of being charged with fraud. However, many times the third-party payer simply changes the code to one that has a lower reimbursement. Down coding is when a claim contains a procedure code that is reimbursed at a lower rate than the procedure actually performed on the patient. Healthcare providers do this to avoid the chance that the claim will be held up by the third-party payer.

- **Unbundling.** This occurs when a claim contains separate procedures that should have been grouped into a bundled procedure. A bundled procedure is a group of related procedures that are reimbursed at a single rate. For example, removal of a gallbladder involves surgery but also preexamination and postexamination. The claim shows the bundled procedure and not the procedures related to the surgery.

3. Dumb Mistakes

Claims are frequently denied because of rookie mistakes that even seasoned professionals make when they are in a rush to file a claim with a third-party payer. Rookie mistakes are normally caused by failing to double-check the claim before filing it. Here are the most common of these.

- **Typographical errors.** Typing errors result in incorrect information appearing on a claim. Take time to proofread the claim to identify and then correct keyboarding errors.

- **Omissions.** Failing to include basic information on a claim causes the third-party payer to immediately reject the claim. Make sure the claim has procedure codes, diagnosis codes, dates of service, the policy identification number, the healthcare provider's tax identification number, and the complete and correctly spelled names of the policyholder and the patient.

- **Identification on support documents.** Each document submitted in support of the claim must have the patient's and policyholder's full, correct name and the policy number.

- **Intact claim form.** Information must appear within the proper area of a printed claim form and the bar code on the claim form must be unobstructed. An improperly positioned claim form in the printer is the most common source of information being misaligned on the form. Stapling over the bar code is a reason why a bar code reader is unable to properly read a claims form.

4. Red Flags

Anything suspicious about a claim or a series of claims involving the same healthcare provider might cause an insurer to turn the matter over to investigators. Each insurer has its own factors that trigger an investigation; however, here are some that are bound to catch insurers' attention.

- **Undocumented procedure.** Procedures that appear on a claim must have supporting documentation. Furthermore, the documentation must provide the reason for the treatment. Missing supporting documentation might lead the insurer to question whether or not the patient received the procedure.

- **Double billing.** Each item on the claim must coincide with the treatment received by the patient. Any items that appear more than once on a claim need to be explained; otherwise the insurer might consider it double billing.

- **Unnecessary procedures.** Each procedure must be justified by the patient's diagnosis according to generally accepted medical practice. The healthcare provider must include a rationale for performing a procedure that is not normally performed based on the patient's diagnosis. Failure to include the rationale on the claim could lead the insurer to suspect that the procedure was performed simply to increase reimbursements.

- **Itemizing fees.** Charges for items used in a procedure are normally bundled with the fee for the procedure and should not appear individually on the claim. When they do, the insurer might suspect the healthcare provider of a form of double billing.

5. The Penalty for Coding Errors

Most coding errors don't result in an investigation. Instead other consequences occur whenever a claim doesn't conform to the insurer's policies such as denial of the claim, and as a result the healthcare provider is not reimbursed for treating the patient. An invoice is then sent directly to the patient.

An insurer may request the healthcare provider to submit a corrected claim if errors are detected in the original claim. Reimbursement is delayed until the corrected claim is processed, and as a result the practice or healthcare facility's cash flow is disrupted.

Another alternative is for the insurer to reimburse less than the claim amount if the coding error is apparent and the correction would lead to a lower reimbursement. This avoids unnecessary delays if the insurer's adjustment to the claim is correct. However, the healthcare provider might disagree and challenge the adjustment (see Chapter 9).

Depending on the type of error, the insurer might impose a financial penalty on the healthcare provider, which is deducted from the reimbursement. For example, this might happen if the claim is filed past the filing deadline imposed by the insurer.

A more severe consequence is for the insurer to refuse to do business with the healthcare provider. Many healthcare providers reach an agreement with the insurer whereby the insurer sends the healthcare provider patients and in return the healthcare provider lowers his fees for those patients. Once the relationship is severed, the insurer treats the healthcare provider as he would treat any other healthcare provider or simply refuses to accept claims directly from him. When this happens, the healthcare provider invoices patients directly and the patient submits claims to the insurer.

If coding errors are intentional in an effort to increase reimbursement, then the healthcare provider is at risk for losing privileges at healthcare facilities, losing her medical license, and facing criminal charges that could lead to a prison sentence.

CASE STUDY

CASE 1

The manager of a large medical group is experiencing an increase in billing and coding errors that have resulted in decreased or delayed reimbursements leading to a decline in revenue for the practice. The manager asks you, the medical billing and coding professional, the following questions. What is the best response?

QUESTION 1. What happens when the medical insurance specialist assumes that the healthcare provider administered standard treatment to the patient when that treatment wasn't administered?
ANSWER: This is called *assumption coding* and error is easily picked up by the third-party payer's claims processing system, which automatically withholds reimbursement until the healthcare provider supplies supporting documents.

QUESTION 2. Why are claims rejected because of improper documentation?
ANSWER: Each claim must be supported by proper documentation to reinsure the insurance company that the stated treatment was administered. Improper documentation, such as inaccurate or incomplete documents, causes the insurer to reject or withhold reimbursements.

QUESTION 3. Why are claims rejected when we reconstruct the documentation to support a previous claim?
ANSWER: Reconstructing documentation happens when supporting documentation is re-created or existing documentation is altered to support a claim submitted to a third-party payer. Altering documents exposes the healthcare provider to civil and criminal charges of fraud.

QUESTION 4. What are problems with up coding and down coding?
ANSWER: Up coding occurs when the claim contains a procedure code that is reimbursed at a higher rate than the procedure actually performed on the patient. Up coding exposes the healthcare provider to an investigation and risk of being charged with fraud. However, many times the third-party payer simply changes the code to one that has a lower reimbursement. Down coding is when a claim contains a procedure code that is reimbursed at a lower rate than the procedure actually performed on the patient. Healthcare providers do this to avoid the chance that the claim will be held up by the third-party payer.

FINAL CHECKUP

1. **Why are practitioners concerned about medical coding and billing errors?**

   A. Errors can be corrected and the revenue stream restored.

   B. Errors increase claim processing.

   C. Errors cause increase of revenue to the practice. Any increase of revenue has nearly the same effect as a patient who is bleeding. As the stream slows, the medical practice or healthcare facility slowly dies.

   D. Errors cause disruption of revenue to the practice. Any disruption of revenue has nearly the same effect as a patient who is bleeding. As the stream slows, the medical practice or healthcare facility slowly dies.

2. **Errors in medical coding and billing also affect patient relations because**

   A. All charges rejected by the insurer are paid by the patient.

   B. The patient may be charged amounts not reimbursed by the insurer as a result of medical billing and coding errors.

   C. The insurer may be charged amounts not reimbursed by the patient as a result of medical billing and coding errors.

   D. The patient may refuse to pay anything except the co-pay.

3. **Besides affecting a practice cash flows and patient relations, what else can happen when medical billing and coding errors occur?**

   A. The practitioner may lose respect from colleagues.

   B. The practitioner may be dropped by the insurer.

   C. The patient may be dropped by the insurer.

   D. Medical billing and coding errors can lead to an investigation by regulators or law enforcement agencies. An innocent mistake might be taken as an evidence of possible fraud.

4. **Mismatch coding occurs when an element of the claim is not consistent with other elements, such as the gender is coded as male for a diagnosis of a hysterectomy.**

   A. True

   B. False

5. **Unbundling occurs when a claim contains separate procedures that should have been grouped into a bundled procedure.**

   A. True

   B. False

6. **A claim that does not adhere to policies of the insurer is called**

   A. Compliance

   B. Bounding

    C. Noncompliance

    D. Fraud

7. **Any items that appear more than once in a claim may be considered double billing.**

    A. True

    B. False

8. **Itemizing fees may be considered**

    A. Mismatch coding

    B. Reconstruction of documentation

    C. Omissions

    D. Double billing

9. **All medical coding and billing errors can be eliminated.**

    A. True

    B. False

10. **An investigator reviewing a claim may not examine other claims to determine if a pattern of fraud exists.**

    A. True

    B. False

CORRECT ANSWERS AND RATIONALES

1. D. Errors cause disruption of revenue to the practice. Any disruption of revenue has nearly the same effect as a patient who is bleeding. As the stream slows, the medical practice or healthcare facility slowly dies.
2. B. The patient may be charged amounts not reimbursed by the insurer as a result of medical billing and coding errors.
3. D. Medical billing and coding errors can lead to an investigation by regulators or law enforcement agencies. An innocent mistake might be taken as evidence of possible fraud.
4. A. True.
5. A. True.
6. C. Noncompliance.
7. A. True.
8. D. Double billing.
9. B. False.
10. B. False.

chapter 9

Strategies for Handling Claim Disputes

KEY TERMS

276 message	Inquiry/Response
277 message	Inactive Policy
Adjudication Process	Inquiry
Apply a Penalty	Level of Care too High
Claim Control Number	No Preauthorization
Claimant	Nonpars
Claims Adjudication	Not Medically Necessary
Clean Claim	Out-of-Network
Down Code the Reimbursement	Procedure Not Covered
Edit	Reconciliation Process
Electronic Funds Transfer (EFT)	Remittance Advice (RA)
Explanation of Benefits (EOB)	Threshold Amount
HIPAA Health Care Claim Status	

1. The Claim Adjudication Process

Medical insurers seem to have the upper hand when dealing with patients and healthcare providers because the insurer determines which procedures are covered by the policy and how much to reimburse the healthcare provider for performing those procedures—or so it seems.

In reality, every claim undergoes an **adjudication process** during which a claims examiner determines whether the claim is covered by the terms of the patient's insurance policy. If the claim is denied, the healthcare provider and the patient can appeal the claim examiner's decision. Some claims shouldn't be appealed, while others must.

Claims adjudication is the comparing of a claim to payer edits and the patient's health plan benefits to verify that the required information is available to process the claim; the claim is not a duplicate; payer rules and procedures have been followed; and procedures performed or services provided are covered benefits, according to Michelle Green in *Understanding Health Insurance,* 11th edition.

Claim adjudication is the process used by a payer to decide whether a claim should be reimbursed. Although each payer has their own multistep process for approving claims, the process is generally the same for all payers.

When the claim is received by the payer, their computer software performs a comprehensive review to discover obvious errors that would prevent the payer from reimbursing the healthcare provider. This step is referred to as an *edit*. Once it's determined that the claim is complete and accurate it is considered a *clean claim*.

To determine whether the claim is clean, the payer's computer software scans the information on the claim to ensure that it contains all the necessary information to process the claim and determines if that information is correct and that the claim conforms to the payers' policies.

For example, the computer software validates the policy number on the claim and determines whether the policy covers the procedures, tests, and other services that appear on the claim based on the policy's master benefit list. Likewise, it determines whether each procedure on the claim is dated and if the date is within the time frame for submitting the claim based on policies established by the payer. Michelle Green and JoAnn Rowell (*Understanding Health Insurance*, 11th edition) suggest that after which a determination is made as to the allowed charges, which is the maximum amount the payer will allow for each procedure or service, according to the patient's policy.

Also, based upon the patient's policy, each procedure is closely examined by the payer's software program to determine if preapproval is required. If so, it looks for corresponding authorization numbers in their data files given to the healthcare provider when the procedure was preapproved.

The computer software also looks for information that doesn't make sense such as a hysterectomy performed on a male patient or procedures listed without fees. All the common errors that were discussed in Chapter 8 are captured during the edit stage of the claims adjudication process.

Claims that fail the edit can be denied outright or forwarded to a claims examiner. A claims examiner is the payer's claims insurance specialist who reviews the claim and decides the appropriate course of action. Let's say the claim is missing information, the claims examiner might ask the healthcare provider to resubmit a corrected claim or additional information for consideration. The resubmitted claim must pass the same computer software edit before moving to the next step in the claims adjudication process.

2. The Medical Review Department

Claims that pass the edit enter the medical review stage of the claims adjudication process that is performed by the payer's medical review department. The medical review department has a team of claims examiners and medical professionals who determine if the patient received appropriate, necessary, and the most cost-effective care from the healthcare provider.

A medical review claims examiner is the first person to review a claim. The examiner doesn't have any clinical experience but is trained to compare an insurance claim form and supporting documents to the terms of the patient's policy and ensure medical necessity.

The examiner makes sure that the patient didn't receive elective, experimental, or unnecessary procedures, which are not normally covered by an insurance policy. Furthermore, the examiner compares the claim with previous claims for the patient to determine whether the patient has reached frequency limits of the policy. A frequency limit sets the maximum number of times the patient will be reimbursed for a medical service.

For example, some policies will reimburse a patient for one routine medical examination per year. Subsequent medical examinations must not be considered a routine examination within the same time frame; otherwise the payer will not reimburse the patient or the healthcare provider.

The examiner also conducts a utilization review if the care was given in a healthcare facility such as a hospital. The objective is to determine whether the healthcare facility was the appropriate place for the care.

The examiner authorizes reimbursement if the policy covers the claim or exercises one of following options if he questions the claim. The examiner can:

- Ask a medical professional (registered nurse or physician) in the claims review department to review the claim. This happens when the examiner feels unqualified to make a determination about the claim.

- Ask the healthcare provider to supply additional information, in the event supporting documents don't provide the rationale for performing a procedure.

- **Down code the reimbursement**. This occurs when the examiner feels that the fee for a procedure is higher than the agreed-upon level and the examiner either lowers the reimbursement or changes the code to a lower cost procedure rather than denying the claim.

- **Apply a penalty**. If a healthcare provider violated a clause in an agreement with an insurer, the examiner may impose a penalty, which is reduced from the reimbursement. For example, a penalty is typically imposed if the healthcare provider submitted the claim that has passed the filing deadline.

- **Deny the claim.** Reimbursement is not authorized.

- Forward the claim to the insurer's investigation and audit department. This is done if the examiner suspects that the claim is fraudulent.

Following up on a Claim

With the volume of claims filed each day by a medical practice or healthcare facility, it is critical that the medical insurance specialist keep track of the status of each claim that is in the claim adjudication process in order to ensure timely reimbursements.

An insurer should respond within 14 days from the date the claim is filed. The medical insurance specialist should follow up with the insurer on the 15th day if there isn't a response to the claim.

Some medical management software has an automated claims status request feature that tracks the claims status. It determines outstanding claims and then automatically sends an electronic inquiry to the insurer regarding the status of the claim.

Inquiries and responses about pending claims are made using the HIPAA Health Care Claim Status Inquiry/Response electronic transaction format that is available at most medical practices, healthcare facilities, and insurers.

An **inquiry** is referred to as a *276 message,* and a response is a *277 message.* A request message contains information that identifies the claim in question and the payer's response by using a response code. These are

- **A Acknowledge.** The insurer acknowledges receipt of the claim.
- **E Transmission error.** The message was garbled and needs resending.
- **F Finalized.** The claim is approved.
- **P Pending.** The insurer is waiting for additional information.
- **R Request for more information.** The insurer requests additional information about the claim.

The **HIPAA Health Care Claim Status Inquiry/Response** electronic transaction format is not a substitute for personal contact with the claims examiner and other representatives from the insurer. Medical insurance specialists should develop a rapport with claims examiners who frequently handle their claims.

In doing so, the medical insurance specialist should be familiar with the insurer's policies and schedule for processing claims. She should learn the particulars about each insurer's claims adjudication process and the level of authority each member of the medical review team has to approve a claim. This gives you an idea who on the team needs to sign off on your claim.

Knowing the insurer's adjudication process gives you the opportunity to learn shortcuts through its system that help speed up reimbursements. For example, an insurer may have a telephony system that enables you to send missing or corrected claims information by pressing buttons on your telephone. A telephony system uses buttons on the telephone to interact with computer software (ie, "press 1 for customer service, press 2 if you want to place an order").

Remittance Advice

The results of the claims adjudication process are sent to the healthcare provider as a *remittance advice* (RA). The RA summarizes adjudicated claims submitted by the healthcare provider to the payer.

The RA groups claims by healthcare provider. One RA could have claims for several of the healthcare provider's patients. Likewise, the reimbursement check contains the total amount due to the healthcare provider for all the claims that have been adjudicated.

The insurer sends the patient an **explanation of benefits** (EOB) when the claim is adjudicated. The EOB summarizes all adjudicated claims for that patient. Let's say that the patient visited the healthcare provider three times during the month, each resulting in a separate claim. The summary of all three appears on the EOB if the insurer adjudicates them at the same time.

3. Remittance Advice Confusion

The RA can be confusing because the results of adjudicating several claims appear on one document. Likewise, reimbursements are lumped together into one check. Therefore, it is critical for the medical insurance specialist to carefully compare each claim summarized on the RA, to the claim submitted to the insurer.

Reimbursement is sent along with the RA for claims that have been partially or totally approved by the claims examiner. An explanation appears next to each claim summary explaining why the claim was partially reimbursed. An explanation is also given for claims that have been denied or held pending receipt of missing information or corrected information.

It is imperative that the medical insurance specialist updates the patient's financial records to reflect the claim summary on the RA. Analyze the reason for partial reimbursement or denial of the claim and determine if it is justified. If it isn't, then develop a strategy with the healthcare provider to appeal the adjudication of the claim.

Be aware that the healthcare provider is reimbursed only if the patient assigned the benefits from the insurance policy to the healthcare provider. This is usually a consent form that patients sign before they are seen by the health-care provider. If they did not make this assignment, then the reimbursement is sent to the patient along with the EOB. Under this circumstance, the health-care provider should collect the fee from the patient at the time the services are rendered to the patient. Otherwise the healthcare provider must trust that the patient will use the reimbursement from the insurer to pay the healthcare provider.

4. Explanation of Benefits Confusion

The EOB can be confusing to the patient who might be seeing it for the first time. The patient might view this as a bill from his insurer rather than a sum-mary of services that the insurer reimbursed the healthcare provider.

Complications arise if some or the entire claim is denied because the patient is unexpectedly liable for the expense—and the reason for the denial can be difficult for the patient to comprehend. The patient finds himself in a medical squabble between the insurer and the healthcare provider.

In these situations the patient normally contacts the medical insurance spe-cialist to help him sort through the EOB. The medical insurance specialist should set aside time to explain the EOB, the patient's insurance policy, and why selective services are covered/not covered by the policy.

If possible, the medical insurance specialist should take on the role of an ombudsman who uses her contacts at the insurer to resolve issues in the EOB.

The patient may erroneously believe he came into money when the EOB is accompanied by a reimbursement check, if benefits were not assigned to the healthcare provider. Therefore it is important that the medical billing specialist advises the patient before the services are rendered as well as send them a cor-respondence reminder to sign the reimbursement to the healthcare provider upon receipt.

5. Reviewing a Remittance Advice

An RA must be reconciled against each claim to be sure that the insurer has properly reimbursed the healthcare provider. The reconciliation process also identifies discrepancies that disallowed full reimbursement.

The **reconciliation process** begins by matching each claim on the RA with the claim that was submitted to the payer using the internal claim control number. The **claim control number** is the unique number that the medical insurance specialist assigns to the patient's account which reflects on the claim before submitting it to the insurer for processing.

After locating the claim, verify that the adjudication result on the RA and the claim are the same by comparing the information about the patient and each procedure listed on the claim. This ensures that the claims control number on the RA refers to the correct claim.

Next, compare procedures. The RA should list the same procedures as shown on the claim. Make note of any description. Also compare the reimbursement for each procedure on the RA and to the fee listed on the claim.

Sometimes a claims examiner will disagree with a fee and reimburse at a lower fee or simply deny reimbursement for the procedure. This is evident if the reimbursement on the RA is less than the fee on the claim. In this situation the RA contains an explanation for the reduction or denial.

Note the discrepancy and the explanation. After the reconciliation process is completed, you can discuss all the discrepancies with the healthcare provider. The healthcare provider has the option to accept or disagree with the adjudication of a claim. If the healthcare provider disagrees, then the claim can be resubmitted or appealed to a higher authority with the payer's appeal's division to reconsider the claim for payment or increase reimbursement.

The next step in the reconciliation process is to update the patient's financial records to reflect the result of the adjudication of the claim. It is important that you record the status of each procedure in the patient's record as reimbursed, accepted adjustment to the claim, or appealing adjustment to the claim. Place a copy of the RA in the patient's records.

The final step is to deposit the reimbursement check. Large medical practices and healthcare facilities use **electronic funds transfer** (EFT) to receive reimbursements from payers. Through EFT an insurer electronically deposits the reimbursement into the healthcare provider's bank account.

Since the payer doesn't issue a check, there isn't a float period during which the check clears. Instead, reimbursements deposited using EFT are available for immediate use by the healthcare provider.

6. Handling Exceptions

In a perfect world a claim submitted to an insurer is fully reimbursed. However, this is not always the case in the real world because claims are either partially reimbursed or denied because of a variety of reasons that are stated on the RA.

When this happens, the medical insurance specialist must immediately determine the reason and take steps to rectify the situation. Many times the claims form has missing or incomplete information that caused the claims examiner to deny the claim. Correcting the claim and resubmitting it to the insurer easily address this problem.

When doing so, make sure that the revised claim is complete before sending it back to the insurer. Occasionally there is more than one mistake that caused the claim to be denied. A medical insurance specialist may be in a rush to resubmit the claim and correct only one problem with the claim, resulting in the claim being denied a second time.

Claims are also denied for other reasons besides errors on the claim such as when the medical review team decides that the procedure was unnecessary or the procedure is ineligible for coverage based on the patient's policy.

If the denial of the claim or a procedure is reasonable, then the healthcare provider may accept the adjudication and either absorb the expense or send the patient an invoice.

However, some reasons given for denial are subjective based on the interpretation of the patient's policy and medical records. This gives the healthcare provider a foundation to appeal the denial (see the following section).

The medical insurance specialist should keep a denial log. A denial log is a notebook that lists reasons why claims were partially or fully denied, and is used to develop procedures that reduce the likelihood that the insurer will deny future claims.

Let's say that after reviewing the denial log the medical insurance specialist notices an unusually large number of claims being returned because of a missing policy number. The medical insurance specialist can institute a new procedure where another person in the office double-checks each claim for key information before the claim is submitted to the payer.

The Appeal

A healthcare provider can request that the insurer to reconsider any claim that has been partially or totally denied by following the insurer's appeals process. The appeals process is the insurer's internal review of the claim examiner's adjudication of the claim.

Only healthcare providers who participate in the payer's program can file an appeal. Those who do not participate—referred to as *nonpars*—are not permitted to appeal. **Nonpars** are expected to collect fees from the patient at the time of service. The patient then files the claim and receives reimbursement from the insurer. A patient then has the right to file an appeal.

The healthcare provider or the patient who files the appeal is called the *claimant* because they filed a claim with the insurer. A claim financially impacts both the healthcare provider and the patient since the patient is typically liable for fees not reimbursed by the insurer.

It is wise for the healthcare provider to obtain a limited power of attorney from the patient before filing an appeal. A limited power of attorney is a legal document that gives the healthcare provider limited rights to represent the patient in matters related to the claim. It also gives the healthcare provider the right to make decisions for the patient in this regard. This means the patient is bound by whatever settlement is reached between the insurer and the healthcare provider regarding the claim.

In an appeal, the healthcare provider writes a letter that challenges the rationale given by the claims examiner for denying the claim by submitting her own rationale along with supporting documentation justifying the treatment rendered. Therefore, the medical insurance specialist and the healthcare provider must devise an argument that shows the claims examiner made an error.

Sometimes it is difficult to counter the claims examiner's reasoning. For example, the patient's policy might not have been enforced when the patient was treated. It might not be wise to file an appeal in these situations unless the patient proves that the policy was active at that time.

Before appealing, make sure that you have a strong case and review the payer's appeals process carefully; otherwise your appeal may be turned down or delayed because of technical problems rather than on the merits of your argument.

Question the claims examiner before submitting an appeal to clarify his position. You might discover there was a misunderstanding that can be resolved by submitting a corrected claim.

Insurers usually have three levels of appeals. These are known as a *complaint, an appeal,* and *a grievance.* All appeals begin at the complaint level and then proceed through the other levels if the claims examiner's adjudication isn't reversed.

There is a deadline for filing the appeal that begins when the RA is sent to the healthcare provider. Appeals filed after the deadline could be automatically rejected depending on the payer. It is important to know the filing deadline when you receive the RA.

A payer might set a threshold amount for an appeal. A **threshold amount** is a minimum dollar amount that can be appealed. Appeals for an amount below the threshold amount are automatically rejected by the payer and cannot be appealed.

After exhausting all appeals with the payer, the healthcare provider can take the appeal to the government agency that oversees the insurance industry, which is usually the state commissioner of insurance.

Each government agency has its own appeals process. It is very important to follow this process exactly because if the appeal is rejected, an attorney can be hired to take the matter through the courts. Failure to follow the government agency's appeals process might prohibit appealing the agency's decision to the courts.

The Appeals Strategy

Develop a strategy for your appeal. Here are a few techniques used when appealing commonly given rationales for denying a claim.

- **Not medically necessary.** You must prove that the service was necessary. Make sure that the proper diagnosis and procedure codes were used on the claim. Sometimes you can simply review the diagnosis and procedure codes with the healthcare provider to determine whether a more appropriate code can be used based on the patient's report and submit a corrected claim without having to go through an appeal. If the codes are correct, then the healthcare provider must submit a letter to the payer clearly stating the patient's conditions that made this case different from the typical case.

- **Inactive policy.** Ask the patient to supply proof that the policy was active at the time service was given. Proof can be in the form of a letter from the patient's employer that contains all the pertinent information about the policy or a letter from the insurer stating that the policy was active at the time. Submit a copy of the proof to the insurer as part of the appeal. Don't appeal if the original claim was correct and the patient is unable to provide you with proof.

- **Procedure not covered.** Make sure that the claim contains the correct diagnosis and procedure codes. If necessary, send the payer a corrected claim. Ask the patient to supply proof that his policy covers the procedure and then forward this as part of the appeal. If the original claim is correct and the patient cannot provide proof of coverage, then submit supporting documentation such as a narrative detailing the medical necessity of the procedure and requesting a onetime consideration for payment based on the patient's medical circumstance.

- **No preauthorization.** Explain the reason that prevented the healthcare provider from asking for authorization prior to performing the procedure such as a medical emergency. Also supply evidence that the procedure would likely have been approved if the healthcare provider had time to contact the insurer. A convincing argument may assist with restoring full reimbursement and cause the payer to waive penalties for not receiving preauthorization.

- **Level of care too high.** Usually the claim fails to contain sufficient documentation that proved the need to give the patient a higher than normal level of care. The best reply is to supply the additional documentation.

- **Out-of-network.** Although it might be true that the healthcare provider does not participate in the payer's program, a strong argument can be made for reimbursing the healthcare provider if an in-network healthcare provider wasn't available to treat the patient. Explain in the appeal why the patient was unable to stay within network such as an emergency or was traveling at the time she fell ill.

CASE STUDY

CASE 1
You have applied for a position as a medical billing specialist for a large healthcare facility. The manager of the department asks you the following questions about appeal strategies. What is your best response?

QUESTION 1. What must be done if the insurer denies the claim stating that a procedure was not medically necessary?
ANSWER: You must prove that the service was necessary. Make sure that the proper diagnosis and procedure codes were used on the claim. Sometimes you can simply review the diagnosis and procedure codes with the healthcare provider to determine whether a more appropriate code can be used based on the patient's report and submit a corrected claim without having to go through an appeal. If the codes are correct, then the healthcare provider must submit a letter to the payer clearly stating the patient's conditions that made this case different from the typical case.

QUESTION 2. What must be done if the insurer denies the claim stating that a procedure was not preauthorized?
ANSWER: Explain the reason that prevented the healthcare provider from asking for authorization prior to performing the procedure such as a medical emergency.

Also supply evidence that the procedure would likely have been approved if the healthcare provider had time to contact the insurer. A convincing argument may assist with restoring full reimbursement and cause the payer to waive penalties for not receiving preauthorization.

QUESTION 3. What must be done if the insurer denies the claim stating that the provider is out-of-network?
ANSWER: Although it might be true that the healthcare provider does not participate in the payer's program, a strong argument can be made for reimbursing the healthcare provider if an in-network healthcare provider wasn't available to treat the patient. Explain in the appeal why the patient was unable to stay within network such as an emergency or was traveling at the time she fell ill.

QUESTION 4. What must be done if the insurer denies the claim stating that the level of care is too high?
ANSWER: Usually the claim fails to contain sufficient documentation that proved the need to give the patient a higher than normal level of care. The best reply is to supply the additional documentation.

FINAL CHECKUP

1. **What are nonpars?**
   A. Healthcare providers who participate in the payer's program.
   B. Healthcare providers who do not participate in the payer's program.
   C. The appeals process.
   D. Claim examiner.

2. **What is electronic funds transfer (EFT)?**
   A. The system used to appeal reimbursement claims.
   B. The system used to submit reimbursement claims.
   C. Transfer of reimbursements directly into the healthcare provider's bank account.
   D. The system used by insurers to assess reimbursement claims.

3. **What is the reconciliation process?**
   A. Assignment of the claim control number.
   B. The process of matching a claim on the remittance advice (RA) with claims submitted to the insurer.
   C. Making sure the claim control number hasn't been already used.
   D. Resolving differences among practitioner and patient.

4. Down code reimbursement is when the examiner lowers the reimbursement or changes the code to a lower cost procedures rather than denying the claim.
   A. True
   B. False

5. A penalty can be applied if the healthcare provider violated a clause in an agreement with the insurer.
   A. True
   B. False

6. What is a 276 message?
   A. A denial
   B. A response
   C. An approval
   D. An inquiry

7. An F response code means that the claim is approved.
   A. True
   B. False

8. An explanation of benefit (EOB) is
   A. Sent by the insurer to the patient when the claim is adjudicated.
   B. Sent by the practitioner to the patient when the claim is adjudicated.
   C. Sent by the insurer to the patient when the claim is denied.
   D. Sent by the insurer to the practitioner when the claim is denied.

9. Claims that pass the edit enter the medical review stage of the claims adjudication process that is performed by the payer's medical review department.
   A. True
   B. False

10. An insurer should respond within 14 days from the date that the claim is filed. The medical insurance specialist should follow up with the insurer on the 15th day if there isn't a response to the claim.
    A. True
    B. False

CORRECT ANSWERS AND RATIONALES

1. A. Healthcare providers who participate in the payer's program.
2. C. Transfer of reimbursements directly into the healthcare provider's bank account.

3. B. The process of matching a claim on the RA with claims submitted to the insurer.
4. A. True.
5. A. True.
6. D. An inquiry.
7. A. True.
8. A. Sent by the insurer to the patient when the claim is adjudicated.
9. A. True.
10. A. True.

chapter 10

Medical Transportation

LEARNING OBJECTIVES

1. Transporting Patients
2. Vehicle and Crew Requirements
3. Reasonableness and Medical Necessity
4. Ambulance Condition Codes
5. BLS and ALS Transportation
6. Selecting the Correct Condition Code
7. Transport Indicators

KEY TERMS

Acute Medical Care
Advanced Life Support Ambulance
Ambulance Dispatch Centered
Basic Life Support Ambulance
C5 Transport Indicator
Condition-Based Coding
Diagnosis Code
Emergency Condition Nontraumatic
Emergency Condition Traumatic
Emergency Response
Emergency Transportation

Medical Necessity
Narrative Comment Field
Nonemergency Conditions
Nonemergency Transportation
Nonemergency Transports
Non-Physician Provider Code
Transport Indicator C2 Interfacility
   Transport
Transport Indicator C4 Medically
   Necessary Transport
Transport Indicators

1. Transporting Patients

Patients who are unable to come themselves to the healthcare facility are transported by other means. Transportation is divided into two groups: emergency transportation and nonemergency transportation.

Emergency transportation typically includes emergency medical service (EMS) providers in the form of a ground or air ambulance. **Nonemergency transportation** includes wheelchair vans, taxi cabs, automobile, and buses. Health insurers typically reimburse for medical transportation services if required by the patient's medical condition.

Medical transportation services are billed separately from other medical services such as those generated by hospitals and practitioners. Billing for medical transportation requires **non-physician provider codes,** specifically ambulance codes found in the Ambulance section of the *HCPCS Level II* code book.

Ambulance services are covered under Medicare Part B under the following situations:

- The patient was transported by an approved ambulance service.

- Other modes of transportation were contraindicated because of the patient's medical condition.

- Transportation occurred from the origin and destination that were covered by Medicare. For example, the patient was transported to the nearest appropriate hospital. The patient is transported from a skilled nursing facility to the nearest available healthcare facility that can provide care that is not available at the skilled nursing facility. Transportation from a skilled nursing facility to home is also covered.

- All services are reasonable and medically necessary.

Not all medical transportation is covered especially if less expensive transportation was available. For example, if ground transportation was medically sufficient, then air transportation isn't covered. When basic life support is sufficient, advanced life support isn't covered. If it is more economical to send a patient home in a taxi, then ambulance transportation isn't covered.

2. Vehicle and Crew Requirements

Reimbursement for medical transportation is dependent on the transportation vehicle and the qualifications of the crew aboard the vehicle. The vehicle must be designed and equipped to provide **acute medical care** while transporting patients to a healthcare facility. Equipment includes a stretcher, oxygen, linens, and emergency supplies that are specified by local and state authorities. In addition, the vehicle must have emergency lights and sirens and telecommunication equipment that enable the vehicle to respond to emergencies and communicate with emergency command centers.

There must be at least a two-member crew on the vehicle at all times when transporting a patient. Crew qualifications depend on whether or not the vehicle is designed for basic life support or advanced life support.

A **basic life support ambulance** requires at least one crew member to be a certified emergency medical technician. An **advanced life support ambulance** requires that one member of the crew to be a certified paramedic, able to perform advanced life support care before and during transportation.

3. Reasonableness and Medical Necessity

Ambulance transportation is reimbursed only if the service is medically necessary and reasonable. An insurer may deny a claim if the insurer deems that transportation was unreasonable based on a pattern of uneconomical practices or where costs are excessive. This may occur even if the patient's condition required ambulance transportation.

Transportation claims that are commonly denied are claims for the use of advanced life support transportation when the patient's condition warranted basic life support transportation. The insurer may approve reimbursement for basic life support transportation although the advanced life support transportation was used to transport the patient to the hospital.

Medical necessity is interpreted as transportation that is necessary so not to endanger the patient's health as determined by the patient's medical condition at the time of service. For example, advanced life support transportation is not a medical necessity for a patient who is wheelchair-bound but otherwise stable. The patient could be effectively transported by a wheelchair van or other types of nonemergency transport.

Use caution when coding for transportation. Make sure you know if the transport service was for an emergency or nonemergency. An **emergency response** is responding immediately with a basic life support ambulance or advanced life support ambulance as a result of a call to the police, to emergency center, or otherwise communicated to the ambulance transport. The ambulance arrives quickly to the patient's location. **Nonemergency transports** are scheduled transports.

4. Ambulance Condition Codes

Claims for ambulance transport must contain codes that describe the patient's symptoms or injury to indicate that ambulance transport was medically necessary. Coding must represent the information that the **ambulance dispatch center** received as part of the initial call. This is the information that is used to determine the level of transport services required to care for the patient. You can use the patient care documentation written by the Emergency Medical Technician (EMT) or paramedics to support the need for the ambulance and related treatment.

All reimbursements for ambulance service require the assignment of a diagnosis code. The diagnosis code is based on patient care documentation from the ambulance services and does not require tests and supportive documentation to support a definitive diagnosis by a practitioner.

The diagnosis code on the claim for reimbursements for ambulance services is likely different from the final diagnosis arrived at by the practitioner after extensive assessments and testing. This is fine because the diagnosis code for ambulance service is based on the presenting signs and symptoms assessed by the EMT or paramedic. The objective is to support the medical necessity to transport the patient by ambulance or by other means.

The level of ambulance service is determined by two factors:

- The time the communication center received the call for the ambulance.
- The time that the EMT or paramedics encounter the patient.

Condition-based coding is used to submit a claim for transportation. During the conversation between the communication center and the person requesting the ambulance, the communication center determines the patient's condition based on the caller's information. The communication center then determines to dispatch a basic life support ambulance, advanced life support ambulance, or other transportation.

The EMT or paramedics reassess the level of transportation once they arrive on the scene and determine whether a different level of ambulance transportation is necessary or whether the appropriate transportation was dispatched to the scene.

Generally, if the patient's reported condition was such that advanced life support is necessary and a qualified advanced life support ambulance and crew arrived at the scene, then it is assumed that the advanced life support ambulance was medically necessary. This is true even if the paramedics determine that no advanced life support is necessary.

There are three general groupings of conditions. These are emergency conditions traumatic, emergency conditions nontraumatic, and nonemergency conditions. An *emergency condition traumatic* is a condition where the patient experiences trauma such as a motor vehicle accident. *Emergency condition nontraumatic* is a condition where the patient has a medical emergency, but no trauma occurs such as a patient experiencing chest pains. *Nonemergency condition* is a routine, usually scheduled transportation.

Most claims require one condition code that most closely reflects why the patient required the ambulance and reflects the patient's symptoms identified by the EMT and paramedic. However, you should include two condition codes. One condition code that reflects the patient's condition reported to the communication center and the other reflecting the patient's condition reported by the EMT or paramedic. This distinction becomes important if the communication center dispatched advanced life support and the paramedics determined basic life support transportation are necessary.

5. Basic Life Support and Advanced Life Support Transportation

Always use the **C5 transport indicator** on claims where basic life support ambulance was used to transport a patient who requires advanced life support. This occurs when the call to the communication center indicates that advanced life support is required but only a basic life support ambulance is available to respond to the call. At the scene, the EMT documents that the patient's condition requires advanced life support.

The C5 transport indicator alerts the insurer that there is a discrepancy between the patient's documented condition by the communication center and EMT and the use of the basic life support ambulance. The insurer will likely process the claim quicker if the C5 transport indicator is not used.

Reimbursement will only be for the basic life support ambulance and not for the advanced life support ambulance. Any intent to submit a claim for advanced life support transportation when the patient received basic life support transportation can be considered fraud.

6. Selecting the Correct Condition Code

Choosing the correct condition code for reimbursement for ambulance transportation can be challenging because the patient's condition may be described differently by the communication center, the EMT/paramedics, and the practitioner who treats the patient.

You should choose one condition code that most accurately describes the patient's condition as represented by a condition that appears in the official medical conditions list. You could place additional information about the patient's condition in the **narrative comment field**; however, the medical conditions list is fairly complete and probably contains the code that represents the patient's condition.

There are occasions when you should provide additional supporting documents and add comments in the narrative comment field to assist adjudication of the claim by the insurer. These situations are:

Transport Indicator C2 interfacility transport to indicate that services were not available at the originating facility and therefore the patient had to be transported to a different facility. You need to include the patient's condition to explain the reason the ambulance was required to transport the patient.

Transport Indicator C4 medically necessary transport to indicate that the patient was not transported to the nearest facility. Make sure that you explain the reason for bypassing the closest facility in the narrative comment field.

Table 10–1 contains a description of columns in the medical condition list.

The Ground Ambulance Services section in the Medicare Claims Processing Manual contains the ambulance fee schedule. Ground ambulance services include land and water transportation. There are also categories of air ambulance service. Fees are based on the patient's condition and not the ambulance used for transportation. Mileage must be calculated.

TABLE 10–1 Columns in the Medical Condition List	
Column	Description
1	ICD10 code that describes the patient's condition.
2	A general description of the patient's condition.
3	A specific description of the patient's condition.
4	Description of the appropriate level of service required by the patient's condition.
5	Comments regarding the patient's condition.
6	HCPCS codes associated with the patient's condition.

Table 10–2 contains a list of modifiers and Table 10–3 contains a list of specialty modifiers for ambulance transportation that are used to describe the patient's service. Modifiers are used to identify the origin and destination of the transport.

Table 10–4 contains ground ambulance service codes that describe ground transportation used to transport the patient. Service codes for advanced life support assumes that advanced life support assessment is defined as an assessment performed by a paramedic that was part of an emergency response and only the paramedics—not EMT—were qualified to perform the assessment. It is important that the patient's signs and symptoms that required advanced life support be documented.

TABLE 10–2 Modifiers for Ambulance Transportation	
Modifier	Description
GY	See the payer's modifier fact sheet for information.
QL	The patient is pronounced deceased after the ambulance is called but before the patient is transported. Ground providers can bill a BLS service along with modifier QL. Air providers can use the appropriate air base rate code with modifier QL. There is no rural allowance or mileage billed.
GM	More than one patient is transported in an ambulance. Details are provided in documentation.
GA	The Advance Beneficiary Notice (ABN) has been provided to the patient.
GZ	The claim is expected to be denied based on medical necessity; however, the ABN was not provided to the patient.

TABLE 10–3 Specialty Modifiers for Ambulance Transportation

Modifier	Description
D	Diagnostic or therapeutic site
E	Residential, domiciliary, custodial facility (other than 1819 facility)
G	Hospital-based ESRD facility
H	Hospital
I	Site of transfer (eg, airport or helicopter pad) between modes of ambulance transport
J	Freestanding ESRD facility
N	Skilled nursing facility
P	Physician's office
R	Residence
S	Scene of accident or acute event
X	Intermediate stop at physician's office on way to hospital (destination code only)

TABLE 10–4 Ground Ambulance Transport Code

Code	Description
A0425	Ground mileage per statute mile.
A0426	Ambulance service, advanced life support nonemergency transport.
A0427	Ambulance service, advanced life support emergency transport.
A0428	Ambulance service, basic life support nonemergency transport.
A0429	Ambulance service, basic life support emergency transport.
A0433	Advanced life support including administration of three or more different medications by IV push/bolus or by continuous infusion excluding crystalloid, hypotonic, isotonic, and hypertonic solutions commonly called *dextrose, normal saline, lactated Ringer*. This code is also used if there was manual defibrillation cardioversion, endotracheal intubation, central venous line, cardiac pacing, chest decompression, surgical airway, interosseous line.
A0434	Specialty care transport of a critically injured patient from one facility to another facility. The patient was attended by one or more health professionals from the specialty area such as critical care nursing. This does not include ventilator-dependent patients unless the patient has emergency signs and symptoms.

TABLE 10–5	Transport Indicator Codes
Code	**Description**
C1	Transportation determined necessary by a physician at the originating facility based upon EMTALA regulations and guidelines. The patient's condition should also be reported on the claim.
C2	Transporting a patient from one hospital to another because the patient required a service that was not available at the originating hospital.
C3	Transport in response to a major incident or mechanism of injury.
C4	Transport but not to the nearest facility. Document why the patient wasn't transported to the nearest facility.
C5	Transport a patient with an advanced life support condition by a basic life support ambulance with no advanced life support services provided.
C6	Advanced life support was appropriate based on local medical dispatch protocols but the patient required basic life support based on assessments made by paramedics when they arrived at the scene. Both advanced life support and basic life support transport codes are necessary for the claim.
C7	An advanced life support ambulance was used because a nonemergent patient required monitoring of continuous administration of medications administered through an intravenous line.

7. Transport Indicators

Transport indicators are codes that describe the transportation rather than describing the patient's condition. Transport indicators are not required for all claims; however, transport indicators provide the insurer with additional information that is helpful in an unusual situation to understand the transportation. Table 10–5 contains transport indicators.

CASE STUDY

CASE 1
The ambulance communication center received a call that a 53-year-old man is having chest pains in a restaurant. The call was placed by someone in the restaurant who did not leave a name or contact information. The ambulance dispatched an advanced life support ambulance to the scene. The paramedics determined that the patient was experiencing indigestion. The patient's vital signs and electrocardiogram were normal. The patient at first refused to be taken to the hospital but later agreed. The emergency department's practitioner diagnosed the patient as having indigestion. What is your best response to the following questions?

QUESTION 1. Can a claim be submitted for advanced life support transportation?
ANSWER: Yes, because based on the information provided by the caller to the ambulance communication center it is reasonable to believe that the patient was having symptoms of a heart attack, which requires advanced life support transportation.

QUESTION 2. Do you expect the claim to be denied because the emergency department practitioner's diagnosis did not require advanced life support transport?
ANSWER: No, because the claim is based on the information received by the ambulance communication center. It is common to have sharp disagreements between the ambulance communication center's understanding of the patient's condition and the practitioner's diagnosis because information about the patient's condition is evolving in an emergency.

QUESTION 3. How would you classify the patient's condition?
ANSWER: The patient had an emergency condition nontraumatic because the patient did not show any signs of trauma.

QUESTION 4. What ground ambulance transport code would you use for this claim?
ANSWER: A0427 Ambulance service, advanced life support emergency transport.

FINAL CHECKUP

1. **How do you define a nonemergency transport?**
   A. Transport determined by the EMT when arriving at the scene.
   B. Nontrauma patient.
   C. Scheduled transport.
   D. Trauma patient.

2. **A paramedic staff ambulance is likely what kind of ambulance?**
   A. Basic life support.
   B. Advanced life support.
   C. Trauma ambulance.
   D. Nontrauma ambulance.

3. **How do you define medical necessity?**
   A. Transportation that is not necessary so not to endanger the patient's health as determined by the patient's medical condition at the time of service.
   B. Transportation that is necessary so not to endanger the patient's health as determined by the police department at the time of service.

C. Transportation that is necessary so not to endanger the patient's health as determined by the patient at the time of service.

D. Transportation that is necessary so not to endanger the patient's health as determined by the patient's medical condition at the time of service.

4. **Ambulance service is not covered by Medicare Part B.**

A. True

B. False

5. **Only the practitioner's diagnosis of the patient determines whether or not ambulance transport is a medical necessity.**

A. True

B. False

6. **What is used to determine the level of transport services required to care for the patient?**

A. The insurer.

B. The medical diagnosis made by the practitioner.

C. Information that the ambulance dispatch center received as part of the initial call.

D. Only information provided by the patient.

7. **Condition-based coding is used to submit a claim for transportation.**

A. True

B. False

8. **When would you use the C2 transport indicator?**

A. Services were not available at the originating facility and therefore the patient had to be transported to a different facility.

B. When the patient refused transportation.

C. When transporting a patient from an accident scene to the hospital.

D. When transporting a patient from the hospital to the patient's home.

9. **Never use the narrative comment field.**

A. True

B. False

10. **Transport indicators describe the patient's condition rather than the transportation.**

A. True

B. False

CORRECT ANSWERS AND RATIONALES

1. C. Scheduled transport.
2. B. Advanced life support.
3. D. Transportation that is necessary so not to endanger the patient's health as determined by the patient's medical condition at the time of service.
4. B. False.
5. B. False.
6. C. Information that the ambulance dispatch center received as part of the initial call.
7. A. True.
8. A. Services were not available at the originating facility and therefore the patient had to be transported to a different facility.
9. B. False.
10. B. False.

chapter **11**

Medical Practice

KEY TERMS

Adverse Side Effect	Loading Dose
American Medical Association	Meaningful Use
Bioavailability	Metabolism
Bundled Payment Model	National Patient Safety Goals
Center for Medicare and Medicaid	One Time Order
Services	Onset
Centers for Disease Control (CDC)	Peak
Core Measures	Primary Effect
Distribution	PRN Order
Dosage Form	Route
Duration	Routine Order
Excretion	Side Effective
Food & Drug Administration (FDA)	Stat Order
Half-Life	The Joint Commission
Interoperability	Therapeutic Level

1. Behind the Scenes

There are a lot of activities that take place while the patient is waiting to see the practitioner. The patient is unaware of many of these tasks. The patient arrives and registers at the receptionist's desk. Typically, the receptionist asks for the patient's name and then enters the patient's name into the computer to bring up information about the patient, which usually includes information about the patient's most recent health insurer.

The receptionist asks the patient whether there were any changes in the patient's health insurance since the last visit. If the receptionist does not know the patient or if the health insurance has changed, the receptionist will ask to see the patient's medical insurance card. The patient is then asked to electronically sign-in. The signature is automatically sent to the patient's computerized records. The receptionist makes a copy of the patient's health insurance card, gives the original back to the patient and the patient returns to the waiting room.

The copy of the patient's health insurance card is given to the medical insurance specialist who then reviews the patient's electronic records and the health insurer's reimbursement guidelines. The medical insurance specialist then calls the patient and collects the health insurance co-pay.

While the patient returns to the waiting room, the medical insurance specialist prints and places a copy of the reimbursement guidelines in the patient's record that is given to the practitioner. In some offices, all information about the patient is accessed directly from the computer by the practitioner.

Reimbursement guidelines are a document that lists criteria for reimbursements for assessments, tests, and procedures that the practitioner may order or perform. The practitioner uses reimbursement guidelines as a reference when assessing the patient to ensure that the health insurer will reimburse the practitioner.

The practitioner electronically documents the visit. Some practitioners may document on paper and other staff members may enter the information into the computer. The medical insurance specialist then reviews the reimbursement guidelines and the practitioner's documentation, then prepares and submits the reimbursement forms to the health insurer.

Hospitals

A patient either has a scheduled admission to a hospital or is brought to the emergency department in crisis. A patient who is scheduled to be admitted to the hospital will meet with the admission staff who collects information about the patient and the patient's health insurer. The patient is assigned a medical record number, if one hasn't already been assigned from a previous visit, and a visit identification number. A medical record number uniquely identifies a patient. A visit identification number uniquely identifies a visit to the hospital for the patient.

The patient signs the appropriate admission forms, given an identification bracelet, and then is wheeled to the medical floor where the nursing staff gets the patient settled on the unit.

Typically, information about the patient is passed along to a case manager. A case manager is a staff member who coordinates the patient stay with hospital staff, practitioners, laboratories, and health insurer. It is the case manager's responsibility to ensure that the patient's healthcare team adheres to reimbursement guidelines and standards of care imposed by the hospital.

A patient who visits the emergency department is usually in crisis—and has no plans of going to the hospital. Within minutes of arrival, the admission staff will gather information about the patient either from the patient or from people who accompanied the patient to the hospital.

The admission staff will look up the patient in the hospital computer system. If the patient was previously treated in the hospital, his/her record will appear in the computer along with his/her medical record number. If this is the first encounter, no records will appear and the admission staff will assign the patient a medical record number and enter patient information into the computer. The patient will also be assigned a visit identification number.

The patient or a relative will be asked to sign the admitting papers. If the patient is unable to sign, then the healthcare team will continue care to stabilize the patient under the presumption that that patient would want to be stabilized.

The patient is then assessed by the triage nurse. The triage nurse performs the initial assessment, identifies the current problem, and records the patient's current and historical medical information. The triage nurse determines the order in which the patient will be seen by the practitioner compared with the condition of other patients in the emergency department.

While the healthcare team is focused on the patient, the case manager or the medical insurance specialist is coordinating activities with the patient's health insurer to determine reimbursement guidelines and co-pays. Reimbursement guidelines are shared with the practitioner.

The goal for many emergency departments is for every patient to be seen by a practitioner within 20 minutes of arrival. The practitioner's goal is to stabilize the patient and then refer the patient to follow-up care.

The patient should be stabilized and discharged within 120 minutes. If the patient is going to be discharged with follow up with the patient's primary-care practitioner. The patient should be discharged from the emergency department and sent to an inpatient unit for follow-up by a hospitalist (practitioner who cares for inpatients) within 220 minutes.

Hospital expenses begin once the patient arrives at the hospital and continues until the patient is discharged.

2. A Visit With a Practitioner

A visit with a practitioner begins with expectations. In the back of the patient's mind, he/she likely hopes that the practitioner can fix what is wrong with the patient. Likewise, the practitioner might be thinking, I hope you have something that I can fix. This might sound strange but the reality is that some practitioners have built a skillset on diagnosing and treating a specific set of disorders. For example, a cardiologist focuses on treating cardiovascular disorder and a pulmonologist treats lung disorders. If a patient presents with a disorder outside the practitioner's skillset, then the practitioner refers the patient to an appropriate practitioner.

The Assessment

After speaking with the patient for a few minutes, the practitioner performs an assessment of the patient to identify what is likely causing the problem. The assessment begins by the practitioner asking the patient to describe how the patient knows that something is wrong. The patient responds by describing symptoms such as nasal congestion and a cough. The practitioner then performs a physical assessment looking for signs of a disorder.

The practitioner follows one of several common assessment methodologies to assess the patient's condition. These include the following:

- **ABCDE**
  - **Airway.** Does the patient have blockage of the airway?
  - **Breathing.** Does the patient have problems breathing?
  - **Circulation.** Does the patient have problems with his heart or blood vessels?
  - **Disability.** Is there anything preventing the patient from performing normal functions of daily living?
  - **Expose and Examine Patient.** The practitioner then takes a close examination of the patient.
- **SAMPLE**
  - **Signs and symptoms.** The practitioner identifies signs (what the practitioner sees) and symptoms (what the patient reports).
  - **Allergies.** Is the patient having an allergic reaction?
  - **Medications.** Is the patient having a side effect or adverse reaction to medication?
  - **Pertinent past medical history.** Is this a continuous problem related to an existing condition?
  - **Last oral intake and menstruation.** Is the problem related to something the patient ingested recently or related to menstruation?
  - **Events leading up to the current problem**. What the patient was doing when he/she noticed the symptoms?
- **OPQRST**
  - **Onset.** When did the problem start?
  - **Provocation.** What makes the problem worse?
  - **Quality.** How do you feel?

- **Radiation.** Does the pain or discomfort move?
- **Severity.** How bad is the problem?
- **Time.** How long have you had this problem?

Tests

The physical assessment of the patient will usually reveal signs of the underlying problem, which when compared with symptoms reported by the patient will enable the practitioner to arrive at a preliminary diagnosis. Some practitioners will prescribe treatment based on the preliminary diagnosis. Alternatively, the practitioner may require medical tests before treating the patient.

There are many kinds of medical tests such as X-rays, echocardiograms, and electrocardiograms. The most common are blood tests. There are also many types of blood tests; some are grouped together into sets of blood tests commonly referred to as a *panel* such as cardiac panel or liver panel. The results of the blood tests tell the practitioner what parts of the body are working. Table 11–1 shows commonly ordered tests.

TABLE 11–1 Common Tests	
Condition	**Tests and Abnormal Results**
Bleeding	• PT (H): Danger 27 • INR (H); PTT (H): Danger 68 • Platelet (L): Danger <37,000 or >910,000
Kidneys	• Creatinine (H); BUN (H) • Output: 1 mL/kg/h to 30 mL/h • Sp Gravity: (H: dehydrated) (L: overhydrated)
Pancreas	• Amylase: H • Lipase: H
Inflammation	• WBC normal: 5,000-10,000 • WBC danger: <2,000 or >25,000 • ESR (H): Inflammation • Neutrophils (H): Bacterial infection/inflammation • Eosinophils (H): Parasitic infection; Basophils (H): Leukemia • Lymphocytes (H): Viral; Monocyte (H); Globulin (H)
Immune system	• CD4+ (L)

(Continued)

TABLE 11–1 Common Tests (*Continued*)	
Condition	**Tests and Abnormal Results**
Anemia	• Hct: L H • Hgb: L • TIBC: L • Transferrin: H • Iron: L • Ferritin: L • RBCs: L
Malnutrition	• Albumin: H • Prealbumin: H
Dehydration	• Hct: H • Hgb: H • Albumin: H • RBCs: H
Liver	• Albumin: L • ALT: H • AST: H • T bilirubin: H • Dir bilirubin: H; bile duct • Indirect bilirubin: H; liver section blocked
Cardiac	• BNP: <100 no heart failure • BNP: 100-300 heart failure • BNP: >900 severe heart failure • CPK-MB: 0-7% no MI (3-6 h MI) • Troponin: >1.4 (3 h to 8 d heart attack)

Abbreviations: ALT, alanine aminotransferase; AST, aspartate aminotransferase; BNP, brain natriuretic peptide; BUN, blood urea nitrogen; ESR, erythrocyte sedimentation rate; H, high; Hct, hematocrit; Hgb, hemoglobin; INR, international normalized ratio; L, low; MI, myocardial infarction; PT, prothrombin time; PTT, partial thromboplastin time; RBC, red blood cell; TIBC, total iron binding capacity; WBC, white blood cell.

Decision

Based on test results and the practitioner's assessment of the patient, the practitioner decides whether she can treat the patient. If so, then the practitioner prescribes medication, therapy, life style changes, or any other treatments that are likely to resolve the patient's problem. If the practitioner is not comfortable treating the patient, then she will tell the patient to see an appropriate practitioner. The practitioner may or may not refer the patient to an appropriate practitioner. The practitioner is careful to follow the health insurer's reimbursement guidelines.

After the Patient Leaves

The practitioner will record assessment, test results, diagnosis, and follow-up care in the patient's chart and provide the medical insurance specialist with information to process reimbursement for the visit.

3. Getting Sick

Our body fixes itself when we are injured, invaded by a microorganism, such as bacteria, or when parts of our body malfunction. At times our body does this quietly without making us realize that anything is wrong. Other times our body lets us know that something is wrong through pain or as a result of the body trying to fix the problem.

Let's say that you ate spoiled food. Nearly immediately, your body detects the problem and goes to work fixing the problem. First you become nauseous followed by cramps in your stomach as your body prepares to void the contents of your stomach. If the food remains for 2 hours or more, then you probably feel cramping in your abdomen as your body stimulates muscles in your intestines and move fluid from other parts of your body to your intestines. You then void your intestines. In both situations, your body is fixing the problem by getting rid of the spoiled food. This is why a practitioner usually doesn't treat vomiting and diarrhea until the body is finished voiding because this is the best way to remove whatever is causing the problem.

Practitioners call this *physiological compensation*. That is, the body is making changes to fix the problem. Some patients who feel sick, would prefer to tough it out, rather than go to a practitioner, giving their body time to address the problem. During this period, the patient helps the body along by conserving energy by staying in bed and taking over-the-counter medication and mom's chicken soup to ease the symptoms.

Symptoms—What We Feel

Symptoms are what we feel, which usually are the effects of our body compensating for the abnormal occurrence. For example, swelling and pain at the site of an injury is caused by the increased flow of blood to the site. Blood provides cells that remove injured tissues and microorganisms that may have entered the body at the site. Also, blood provides increased nutrients so cells can reproduce and repair the damage. Increased blood flow results in swelling and increased temperature at the site. Swelling causes tissue at the site to press against nerves causing pain.

If the body detects an allergen, allergies, then mast cells release histamine that causes blood vessels to be permeable, increasing fluid around the site of the allergen resulting in flushing the allergen from the body. We recognize this as runny nose and eyes, which are common symptoms of allergies. Some patients reverse this symptom by taking antihistamine that reduces the release of histamine and thereby decreasing the flow of excessive fluid—stops runny nose and eyes.

If the body detects a pathogen, a microorganism that causes infection, then among other responses, the hypothalamus increases the body's temperature in an attempt to kill the pathogen. This is why a patient has a high temperature when fighting an infection.

Physiological Reserves—Body's Capability to Fix Self

The body naturally creates physiological reserves that can be used to fix itself when confronted by injury, disease, or malfunction of part of the body. Think of this as having a full tank of gasoline. The body is confronted by pathogens, allergens, and injuries daily. Most times we don't realize it because these are minor episodes and there are sufficient physiological reserves to address the problem.

As long as we take nutrients and the effort for the body to fix itself is minor, we function normally. That is, we are able to replenish our depleted physiological reserves in short time without any effect on our body's function. Think of this as filling the gas tank before running out of fuel.

Physiological Reserves Running Low

During long illnesses or long debilitating injuries, our physiological reserves can run low and reach a point when there aren't enough reserves to fight the illness and repair the injury, and keep us functioning normally. The body is running out of gas.

Naturally the body decides to focus resources on fighting the abnormality taking away resources from functioning normally. The patient then stays in bed, and goes to see the practitioner for help.

Think of this as a car. If the tank has sufficient fuel, the car can chug along with relatively minor engine problems. However, there are times when there is major engine trouble and the car won't run and needs to be attended to by a mechanic.

Supplementing the Physiological Reserves

The practitioner rarely fixes the patient except if the patient requires reconstruction surgery. Instead, the practitioner supplements the patient's physiological reserves with treatment. The treatment continues until the patient's physiological reserves can fix the problem.

Let's say that the patient has a bacterial infection. The patient's immune system can normally combat the bacterial infection. However, the immune system isn't powerful enough to win the battle. After a day or so, symptoms become nearly unbearable and the patient goes to the practitioner for help. The practitioner prescribes an antibiotic. Typically, a double dose is administered first and then the patient continues to take one dose daily for 4 days or so depending on the medication. The bacteria may still be in the patient's body after the medication is stopped; however, the amount of bacteria is probably at the level that the patient's immune system can handle.

4. Medication

There is a tendency to take medication for granted thinking there is a pill that can fix all our problems. This is not true. Medication is a chemical that usually has a basis in nature that has a therapeutic effect on the body. For example, aspirin comes from the white willow bark and morphine comes from the opium poppy. People have been, and still do, use natural ingredients to treat illnesses.

Today pharmaceutical companies create synthetic medications that have the same therapeutic effect as natural ingredients. However, medication is highly regulated by the Food & Drug Administration (FDA). It can take 12 years and $350 million to bring one medication from the laboratory to the market place. Only 1 of 1,000 medications in the laboratory makes to clinical trials.

FDA Approval Process

1. **Animal testing.** The initial test of medication is with animals to determine the safety of the medication. Scientists look at the mechanism of how the drug works in the animal's body.

2. **FDA approves clinical trials.** Once animal testing is completed, the FDA reviews the results and if satisfied that the medication is safe, the FDA approves the medication for clinical trials.

- **Phase 1 Studies—Safety.** The goal of Phase 1 is to identify side effects, how the medication is metabolized, and how the medication is excreted from humans.

- **Phase 2 Studies—Effectiveness.** The goal of Phase 2 is to identify whether the medication works and compares patients who received the medication with patients who received other treatments for the same disorder.

- **Phase 3 Studies—Dosage and Safety.** The goal of Phase 3 is to determine the proper dosage of the medication to achieve the desired therapeutic effect and also determine the effects when the medication is taken with other medication. Another objective is to determine the effects the medication has on different populations.

3. **New drug application (NDA).** When all goals of the clinical trial are met, the pharmaceutical company applies for approval of the new medication.

4. **Approved—Published.** If approved by the Federal Drug Administration, the medication is added to the U.S. Pharmacopeia National Formulary, which is a description of all approved medication in the United States.

Rules of Medication

Before 1938, there was no control over medications. Anyone could practically say anything about "medicine" without having to prove their claim. In 1938, Congress passed the Food, Drug and Cosmetic Act that required medication manufacturers to prove that the medication was safe before it can be sold to the public. Furthermore, manufacturing facilities that made the medication must be inspected by federal inspectors and manufacturers who must determine the safe dose of the medication to prevent patients from being poisoned. In addition, the Act controlled manufacturing of cosmetics and therapeutic devices.

In 1952, Congress passed the Durham-Humphrey Amendment to the Food, Drug and Cosmetic Act that defined a group of medications that could only be purchased by prescription written by a licensed practitioner. Until 1952, anyone could purchase and distribute medication.

In 1962, came the Kefauver-Harris Amendment to the Food, Drug and Cosmetic Act. This amendment focused on labeling and information about the medication. Manufacturers had to use standard labeling for medication containers that lists adverse reactions the patient may experience taking the medication; contraindications that told the patient when not to take the medication; and list of reasons why the medication should not be used.

In the 1960s, there was an upsurge in abuse of certain medications. In 1970, Congress passed the Comprehensive Drug Abuse Prevent and Control Act that categorized controlled substances into a schedule based on potential abuse of the medication. The schedule was divided into five categories:

- **Schedule I.** Medication that is not approved for medical use such as heroin and LSD.
- **Schedule II and III.** Narcotics.
- **Schedule IV and V.** Sedative and barbiturates.

Medication Names

A medication can have three names:

- **Chemical name.** The chemical name is based on the molecular structure such as N-acetyl-p-aminophenol.
- **Generic name.** The generic name is the name given to medication when the medication is approved by the Federal Drug Administration. Any manufacturer of the medication can use the generic name. For example, acetaminophen is the generic name for N-acetyl-p-aminophenol.
- **Brand name.** The brand name is the name given to the medication by the manufacturer who patented the medication. The brand name is used in advertisements. Only the manufacturer who holds the patent for the medication can use the brand name. For example, Tylenol is the brand name for acetaminophen.

Brand Versus Generic Drugs

Brand name medication and its generic equivalent can be confusing to understand since both are practically the same medication. The pharmaceutical company who developed the medication; completed the FDA approval process; and holds the patent for the medication is the only manufacturer that can make the medication. Once the patent expires in 12 years, then another pharmaceutical manufacturer can make the generic version of the medication.

The generic medication has the same active ingredient and the same pharmacological effect as the brand name medication. The generic medication cannot look like the brand name medication.

Generic medication usually costs the patient substantially less than the brand name medication because the generic pharmaceutical manufacturer does not incur research and development cost and the initial expense to bring the medication to market.

Prescriptions Versus Over the Counter

Prescription medication also referred to as *legend medication* is medication that the FDA requires to be dispensed by an order (prescription) written by a practitioner who is licensed by the FDA to prescribe medication. Prescription medications are usually medications that are unsafe for the patient to use unless supervised by a practitioner.

Over-the-counter medications are medications that patients can purchase without having to be under supervision by a practitioner. Medications once available only by prescription are now available over the counter, sometimes in a modified form such as a lower dose.

At times this can be confusing to patients and practitioners. For example, the prescription dose of the anti-inflammatory medication Ibuprofen is 600 mg. The over-the-counter dose is 200 mg. A patient could take three 200 mg pills of Ibuprofen to receive the equivalent of the prescription dose.

Medication and the Body

Pharmacokinetics describes how medication interacts with the body. The first step is the route. The **route** is how the medication gets into the body. These are by mouth, by intramuscular (IM) injection, subcutaneous (SC) injection, intravenous (IV), transdermal (a patch); topical (a thin layer applied on the skin); sublingual (under the tongue); buccal (between gum and cheek); inhalation (aerosol sprays); instillation (nose, eye, ear); suppository (rectal, vaginal); and intradermal (beneath skin). The medication appears in a particular form such as a tablet, capsule, or solution. This is referred to as the *dosage form.*

Once the medication enters the body the medication must be absorbed into the bloodstream, which is referred to as *absorption.* Medication can be absorbed in the intestine, under the tongue (sublingual), by the lungs, or directly injected in the veins (IV). The entire dose of the medication may not be absorbed. A portion of the dose may remain at the site where the medication was administered to the patient. The amount of the dose that is absorbed is referred to as *bioavailability.* Only an intravenous injection delivers 100% of the dose to the patient.

The medication must be converted into the chemical that has desired therapeutic effect. This is referred to as *metabolism.* The **therapeutic effect** is the desired action that the medication has on the body. For example, the therapeutic effect of *Ibuprofen is to reduce inflammation. Many medications are metabolized by the liver, which is referred to as the first pass. If the liver malfunctions, then medication cannot be metabolized and the practitioner orders medication to be administered using a different route such as IM injection.*

The medication must then be transported throughout the body to tissues and organs. This is referred to as *distribution*. Medication is distributed by the cardiovascular system (heart and blood vessels). Each tissue and organ can receive a different dose and the medication can remain in the tissue and organ for varying times. Medication is removed from the body usually through the kidneys and at times in stool. This is referred to as *excretion*.

The practitioner should be concerned if the patient's body is not functioning properly to enable medication to be absorbed, metabolized, distributed, and excreted. Any disruption in this system can result in excess medication being in the patient's body resulting in an adverse side effect.

The practitioner orders medication to be taken at regular intervals in order to maintain a therapeutic level of the active chemical in the bloodstream. Depending on the medication, the practitioner may order an initial higher dose to kick start the treatment. This is referred to as a *loading dose*. For example, the patient may be asked to take two doses of antibiotic the first day of treatment. This increases the therapeutic level in the bloodstream. Medication is identified as having an onset and half-life. **Onset** is the time it takes before the dose has a therapeutic effect. For example, it may take 4 hours before you start to feel better because it takes that long for the medication to reach the therapeutic effect. The length of time of the therapeutic effect is called the medication's *duration*. This is when the medication reaches the highest concentration in the bloodstream, which is called the *peak*. **Half-life** is the period of time when the medication loses the therapeutic effect. The practitioner may tell the patient to take another dose in 12 hours because the medication (half-life) is no longer at a therapeutic level.

A medication can have three effects on the body. These are

- **Primary effect.** The **primary effect** is the desired therapeutic effect. For example, Benadryl decreases histamine that causes a runny nose.
- **Side effect.** A **side effect** is a nontherapeutic effect. For example, Benadryl can cause drowsiness.
- **Adverse side effect.** An **adverse side effect** is an undesirable nontherapeutic effect. For example, in rare cases Benadryl can cause blurred vision and hives.

Medication Action

The therapeutic effect of a medication is determined by how the medication interacts with cells in the body. For example, some medications increase cellular activity and are referred to as *stimulants*. Other medications decrease cellular activities and are referred to as *depressants*.

Still other medications replace essential body compounds such as insulin. These are referred to as *replacement medication*. Medications, such as antibiotics, interfere with cell growth, bacterial cells. These are referred to as *inhibition medication*, and medication such as laxatives are called *irritants* because the medication irritates cells to cause a natural response.

Medication Order

Practitioners order medications in the form of a prescription or as a medication order within a healthcare facility. The medication order must have

- **Medication name.** Medication to be administered.
- **Dose.** The dosage to administer.
- **Frequency.** The number of times the medication is to be administered.
- **Route.** How to administer the medication.
- **Start date/time.** When to begin administration of the medication.
- **End date/time.** When to stop administration of the medication.
- **Parameters.** Measurement, such as blood pressure, heart rate, blood glucose, of when to administer or withhold administration of the medication.
- **Signature.** The practitioner's signature.

Medication orders can be written as a **routine order**, which means that the medication is to be administered at the next schedule time; **PRN** order, which is needed based on specific criteria such as pain or fever; **one time order**, which is a single dose given at a specific time; and a **stat order**, which is one dose to be given immediately.

5. Computerization of Patient Medical Records

In 2004, President George Bush announced in his State of the Union Address that by 2014 the health record of every American will be in an electronic format to avoid dangerous medical mistakes, reduce cost, and improve care. However, the healthcare industry was not quick to embrace this goal primarily because of the cost involved in computerizing health record. Healthcare facilities had to acquire clinical software application, upgrade technology, and rebuild the electronic infrastructure to support electronic health records. Healthcare facilities lacked the financial resources to accomplish this task.

In 2009, Congress passed the American Reinvestment and Recovery Act that provided $19 billion incentive for healthcare facilities and practitioners to use information technology to computerize health records.

In 2010, the Medicare Health Electronic Record Incentive Program established goals for every healthcare facility in the form of **Meaningful Use** requirements. Healthcare facilities and providers must demonstrate that they are using certified electronic health technology to improve the quality and quantity of care in order to receive a portion of the $19 billion incentive approved by Congress. Meaningful Use requirements set progressively increasing goals that eventually will fully automate health records. Failure to comply will eventually result in loss of the incentive and decrease reimbursement of Medicare payments to the healthcare facility and practitioner.

Electronic medical record software applications are provided by one of several major vendors although few healthcare facilities created their own. Vendors ensured the accuracy of data stored in the application and that the application met current and new regulatory requirements.

Healthcare facilities acquired a license to use the vendor's products. Some software products cannot be modified by the healthcare facility. This is similar to you purchasing Microsoft Office. Other software products can be tailored to meet the healthcare facility's requirements. Think of this as purchasing a suit from the rack and having a tailor modify the suit to meet your body contours. However, like a suit, there are limits to what can be modified in the software application.

If tailoring the software doesn't meet the healthcare facility's requirements, then the healthcare facility usually has two options: pay to have the vendor modify the application or request a modification to the vendor's application. Only large healthcare facilities have the resources that pay the vendor to modify their copy of the application. Once modifications are made, then there is a chance that the healthcare facility won't be able to accept regular upgrades without paying for additional modifications. Requesting a change doesn't mean that the change will happen. The vendor typically presents all requested changes to a committee of customers; remember there are many healthcare facilities using the product. If the committee agrees on the change, then the vendor considers including the change in the next release, whenever that happens.

Exchanging patient electronic medical information among healthcare providers is a major challenge facing the movement toward electronic medical records. Each vendor stores patient information in a different format making it difficult to share information electronically. Exchanging electronic information among vendors is called *interoperability*. Standards are being developed to facilitate exchanging patient information electronically.

One such standard is called *Clinical Document Architecture* (CDA) messaging. Vendors are required to format selected patient information into a CDA message. The healthcare facility then electronically sends the CDA message to the healthcare provider/facility that is providing the next level of care to the patient. Think of this as a private email. The existing alternative to the CDA message is called the *Universal Transfer Form*, which is a document containing relevant patient information that is sent on paper to the next level of care facility.

Patients are also able to view their medical records electronically through the Patient Portal. Healthcare providers are required to provide a Web site called a *Patient Portal* that enables the patient to review important pieces of his/her medical record. In addition, some healthcare providers enable patients to make appointments, send inquiries to practitioners, and receive information about disorders/test/medication through the Patient Portal.

6. Business of Medicine

Healthcare is a highly regulated industry both at the federal level and at the state level. In addition, private professional organizations provide oversight to elements of the healthcare industry that greatly influences regulatory authorities.

At the federal level, the **FDA** establishes regulations for the introduction, manufacturing, and administration of medication. Furthermore, the FDA licenses practitioners to prescribe medication.

The **Center for Medicare and Medicaid Services** (CMS) sets reimbursement standards that include guidelines and rates for Medicare reimbursements, which is used by private health insurers to set reimbursement rates for healthcare facilities and practitioners. Furthermore, CMS sets clinical quality measurements and Meaningful Use requirements for all healthcare facilities. Also working at the federal level is the **Centers for Disease Control** (CDC), which collaborates on regulations for controlling diseases.

State regulators issue licenses to health insurers, healthcare facilities, medical schools, and various healthcare practitioners (ie, nurses, nurse practitioners, physicians, physician assistants). Licenses are granted and renewed based on accreditation by private organizations. For example, The **American Medical Association** (AMA) accredits medical schools, certifies physician specialties, and oversees physician license exams. Likewise, **The Joint Commission** accredits hospitals and establishes standards for healthcare facilities through **Core Measures**, which are standard ways to measure a hospital's performance, and **National Patient Safety Goals**, which are procedures that if followed will reduce hospital-acquired diseases and injuries to patients.

Insurer Rules

There are more than 35 major health insurers in the United States and each has multiple health insurance plans that can be tailored to meet the needs of an employer. Employers are a major provider of non-governmental health insurance. The same health insurers typically offer health insurance plans for individuals. Health insurance plans are governed by state and federal regulations that require specific coverage.

Health insurers collectively influence the care and pricing structure of the healthcare industry by the health insurer's rules governing reimbursement. Practitioners and healthcare facilities are free to charge any fee for their service; however, health insurers typically pay what is deemed to be usual and customary fees based on negotiated rates (in-network) with healthcare providers and healthcare facilities or at percentage (80%) of the usual and customary fees for the equivalent service (out-of-network). The patient usually has the option to use an in-network provider and pay a co-pay or use an out-of-network provider and pay 20% of the usual and customary fee.

Health insurers are moving away from a fee-for-service basis where the practitioner is paid a separate fee for each service provided to the patient. In place is a **bundled payment model** where the healthcare provider receives a fix amount of money for a particular group of services. Furthermore, healthcare providers will not receive additional reimbursements if the patient returns within 30 days with the same diagnosis.

Independent Contractors

Healthcare is a fragmented industry where there is confusion over whether a service provided by a healthcare facility is actually provided by the healthcare facility or by an independent contractor. For example, the radiology and pathology departments in a hospital might actually be operated by a firm that has a contract with the hospital. Staff who works in those departments don't work for the hospital. Instead, they work for the contractor. Although they look like hospital employees but they are not employees of the hospital.

Patients learn about this usually when he/she receives separate bills from the independent contractor. For example, it is not unusual to receive a bill from the anesthesiologist for a surgery separately from the surgeon's bill and the hospital bill. Furthermore, the anesthesiologist may not be a part of the health insurer's in-network group of practitioners.

Revenue Streams

A healthcare facility and practitioner receive revenue from several sources. These are

- Health insurer reimbursement. The healthcare facility and practitioner may or may not have a prenegotiated rate with the health insurer.
- CMS. CMS reimburses healthcare facilities and practitioner for providing care to Medicare recipients.
- State government. State government reimburses healthcare facilities and practitioners for Medicaid recipients and patients who are on charity care and have no health insurance.
- Self-pay. A very small amount of revenue is generated from patients who pay out-of-pocket for healthcare.

For Profit Versus Not for Profit

Many healthcare facilities are not for profit although there is a trend for for-profit healthcare facilities coming into play.

A not-for-profit healthcare facility pays no property tax, no income tax, and no sales tax. For this privilege, the facility must use surplus funds—revenue minus expenses—to advance the welfare of the public. Surplus funds must not benefit any individual.

A for-profit healthcare facility pays property taxes, pays income taxes, and pays sales tax. Surplus funds can be reinvested in the healthcare facility, in other investments, or returned to stockholders.

What Is the Real Cost of Healthcare?

Determining the real cost of healthcare is evasive because of the lack of transparency in pricing. The price quoted in the bill is not necessarily the amount received by the healthcare facility. Here are some examples.

- **Same day nonsurgical procedure.** The patient registered in the admissions department of the hospital at 8 AM and was discharged following the procedures at 3 PM. The hospital quoted price was $35,000. The health insurer received a 90% discount bringing the health insurer's portion of the bill to $3,150. The patient's co-pay was $350. It is safe to assume that the $3,500 received by the hospital covered all its expenses plus a surplus.

- **Swab for vaginitis laboratory test.** This is a commonly performed test. The laboratory that conducted the test on the sample quoted a price of $663 but gave the health insurer a $500 discount. The health insurer paid $113.44 and the patient $48.46.

- **Hepatitis C drug.** Hepatitis C is a common viral infection of the liver. A 12-week treatment costs $84,000 in the United States. The same treatment for 24 weeks costs $2,000 in India.

- **Brand drugs:** Catapres is the brand name of a medication that lowers blood pressure. A recent survey found that it costs 40 cents a pill. Whereas, Clonidine the generic bioequivalent of Catapres costs 12 cents per pill.

- **Emergency department visit.** A patient spent 2 hours in the emergency department ($2,609); received one X-ray ($368); and spent overnight for observation in the emergency department ($8,786). The quoted bill was $11,763. The hospital accessed $2,739 as full payment from the health insurer.

- **Gallbladder removal.** Gallbladder removal is one of the most common surgical procedures performed in the United States. It takes 90 minutes to prepare the surgical room, perform the procedure, and clean the room. The turnover between patients is 15 minutes based on a private survey. The hospital billed Medicare $56,000 for inpatient and $12,000 for outpatient. Inpatient is when the patient stayed overnight in the hospital usually to receive additional antibiotics intravenously. Outpatient is when the patient is sent home following a few hours' recovery period. Medicare reimbursed the hospital $10,000 for inpatient and $3,500 for outpatient. The actual expense to the hospital was $1,790 for either inpatient or outpatient.

Reasons for Mergers/Affiliations of Hospitals

The business of healthcare is changing as the focus is trying to give patients more control over their healthcare. Traditional independent practitioners were considered customers of healthcare facilities because the practitioner determined which hospital to recommend to the patient. Likewise, the practitioner referred patients to specialists.

Patients are now selecting the healthcare facility and specialists based on the selection of healthcare facilities and specialists that are in the patient's health insurer's network. Furthermore, healthcare facilities are expending into non-hospital venues, such as urgent care centers, that provide care normally provided by primary-care practitioners. A patient who uses an urgent care center realizes that their electronic health records are available to any practitioner within the hospital's own network of facilities. Care documented at the urgent care center can be brought up at any of the hospital-owned facilities enabling practitioners who work for their hospitals to share information about the patient.

Hospitals also merge and create affiliations with other hospitals. They do so for many purposes. These include to

- Strengthen their position to negotiate rates with health insurers.
- Broaden the offering of services to patients and health insurers. Health insurers prefer to work with one facility that can provide a breadth of services required by patients.
- Reduce competition. Changes in healthcare practice and reimbursements have resulted in excess capacity in some markets.
- Strengthen the healthcare facility's short-term and long-term financial positions by leveraging positive credit rating of the merged or affiliated facility.

Winning Strategy

Some healthcare facilities have developed what they believe is a winning strategy. This includes

- Developing unique profitable services that are not available in their market place.
- Attract a high number of privately insured patients.
- Strict control of expenses.
- Market the healthcare facility to patients.
- Integrate private practices with the healthcare facility.
- Share financial incentives and risks with private practitioners.

Patient Protection and Affordable Care Act

The Patient Protection and Affordable Care Act, commonly referred to as *ObamaCare,* has introduced a new element in the healthcare industry. The underlying current is to move away from employer-based health insurance and toward an open-market health insurance where consumers purchase health insurance directly from health insurers similar to automobile insurance. In theory, this will introduce consumerism where the market place determines the cost of health insurance. Today that cost is buffered by employers who are customers of health insurers.

The Patient Protection and Affordable Care Act introduced the following:

- Preexisting health conditions
  - Past: Increased premium; deny coverage; exclude condition from benefit.
  - Now: No additional charge; must cover preexisting health conditions.
- Preventive care cost
  - Past: Out-of-pocket cost kept people away from care.
  - Now: No out-of-pocket cost; no pay; no minimum deductible.
- Insurance for young adults
  - Past: 18-year-old dropped from parents' health plan with few exceptions.
  - Now: Can remain on parents' health plan up to 26 years.
- Annual and lifetime benefit limits
  - Past: Dollar limits on claims annually and life of policy.
  - Now: No annual and lifetime limits.
- Cost controls
  - Past: Administrative profit taking.
  - Now: Rate increase beyond 10% must be federally reviewed.
  - 80% of premium must pay for actual healthcare.
- Coverage cancellations
  - Past: If insurer found error on insurance application can revoke coverage; force to return paid claims.
  - Now: Can cancel for outright false or incomplete information on an application or not pay premium.
- Right to appeal
  - Past: Insurer refuses to pay claim without explanation.
  - Now: Must explain why claim denied; can appeal to independent third party.

- Minimum coverage
  - Past: No minimum coverage.
  - Now: Required minimum coverage.
- Health insurance
  - Past: Not required with exceptions.
  - Now: Required with exceptions.

CASE STUDY

CASE 1
A newly hired medical insurance specialist is processing reimbursement claims that include among others items of medication. You are asked the following questions. What is the best response?

QUESTION 1. Why did the practitioner order a loading dose?
ANSWER: Depending on the medication, the practitioner may order an initial higher dose to kick start the treatment. This is referred to as a *loading dose.*

QUESTION 2. Why did the practitioner order a generic medication rather than the brand medication?
ANSWER: The generic medication has the same active ingredient and the same pharmacological effect as the brand name medication. Generic medication usually costs the patient substantially less than the brand name medication because the generic pharmaceutical manufacturer does not incur research and development cost and the initial expense to bring the medication to market.

QUESTION 3. Why is this medication ordered as PRN?
ANSWER: PRN indicates that the medication is administered to the patient as needed based on specific criteria such as pain or fever. If the patient doesn't meet the criteria, then the medication is not administered.

QUESTION 4. What is the difference between a stat order and a one-time order?
ANSWER: A one-time order states that a dose of the medication is given once but not necessarily again. A stat order states that a dose of medication must be administered immediately.

FINAL CHECKUP

1. **What does a patient tell a practitioner during a visit?**

   A. Signs

   B. Symptoms

   C. Signs and symptoms

   D. Treatment plans

2. **Why does a practitioner order medical tests?**

   A. To identify symptoms of a disease.

   B. To gather additional objective information about the patient's conditions.

   C. To increase reimbursements.

   D. To reassure the patient about the prescribed treatment.

3. **What are a patient's physiological reserves?**

   A. A form of co-pay.

   B. Medication that is prescribed by the practitioner.

   C. A comprehensive health insurance policy.

   D. The capabilities of the body to repair itself.

4. **All medications had to be prescribed by a licensed practitioner before 1938.**

   A. True

   B. False

5. **Practitioners must be licensed by the Food & Drug Administration to prescribe medications.**

   A. True

   B. False

6. **Meaningful Use is a program that**

   A. Requires healthcare facilities/providers to use paper patient records to better the quality of healthcare given to patients.

   B. Requires healthcare facilities/providers to use technology to better the quality of healthcare given to patients.

   C. Guarantees all patient healthcare records will be computerized.

   D. Guarantees all clinical staff use electronic healthcare records.

7. **CDA messaging is used to share a portion of a patient's healthcare record with another healthcare facility.**

   A. True

   B. False

8. **What is the role of The Joint Commission?**

   A. The Joint Commission accredits hospitals and establishes standards for health-care facilities.

   B. The Joint Commission accredits medical schools.

   C. The Joint Commission oversees physician license exams.

   D. The Joint Commission certifies physician specialties.

9. **Health insurers are moving away from a fee-for-service model.**

   A. True

   B. False

10. **A for-profit healthcare facility pays property taxes, pays income taxes, and pays sales tax.**

    A. True

    B. False

CORRECT ANSWERS AND RATIONALES

1. B. Symptoms.
2. B. To gather additional objective information about the patient's conditions.
3. D. The capabilities of the body to repair itself.
4. B. False.
5. A. True.
6. B. Requires healthcare facilities/providers to use technology to better the quality of healthcare given to patients.
7. A. True.
8. A. The Joint Commission accredits hospitals and establishes standards for health-care facilities.
9. A. True.
10. A. True.

chapter 12

Medical Billing Software Programs and Systems

LEARNING OBJECTIVES

1. Computerization
2. The Network Connect
3. A Computer Program
4. Navigating a Computer Program
5. New Patient Entry
6. The Encounter
7. Posting Payment
8. Patient Statement

KEY TERMS

Bill Type

Computer Network

Computerization

Electronic Envelope

Encounter

Encrypted

Guarantor

Internet Protocol (IP) Address

Medical Management Program

Packet

Patient Statement

Posting the Payment

Router

The Medical Manager

Walkout Receipt

1. Computerization

"But I have the green card from the post office that shows you received our claim!"

This cry is no longer being heard from healthcare providers who computerize patient's medical records and submit electronic claims to insurers. Insurers no longer can say they didn't receive a claim sent by certified mail because the claim is automatically accepted and stored in their computer systems.

Nearly 75% of medical insurance claims and all Medicare claims are processed electronically using a computer program resulting in 98% of those claims being reimbursed within 30 days.

Today medical insurance specialists must be as well versed in medical management software programs as they are in medical insurance.

The medical industry is undergoing a revolution that occurred decades ago in other industries—it is beginning to computerize. Although some hospitals continue to use paper charts, it is now becoming mandatory to computerize all medical records.

Computerization is the process of recording, storing, and retrieving information electronically. It begins with the first encounter with the patient when he/she sits in the waiting room filling out a general information form, a medical insurance form, and a subjective medical history form.

The patient's handwritten forms are transcribed or scanned into a medical management computer program where the information is stored on a computer. Once stored, healthcare providers, medical insurance specialists, and others on the medical team can recall the patient's information using the office desktop computer.

After the healthcare provider examines the patient, the patient's medical records are updated with diagnoses, medical orders, medical tests, and treatments given to the patient. Some healthcare providers are also able to send prescriptions to pharmacies electronically via the Internet.

Maintaining a patient's medical record is a collaborative responsibility. In a hospital, a healthcare provider's medical orders are entered into the hospital's medical management program. The **medical management program** channels the medical order to the appropriate healthcare provider who is responsible for carrying out the order.

The pharmacist receives prescriptions and laboratory technicians receive orders to perform medical tests by checking the medical management program for the latest medical orders. The results of medical orders are then entered into the medical management program and are immediately made available to the healthcare provider—from within the hospital, in his office, or from his home and mobile computer.

2. The Network Connect

A patient's medical information is shared among healthcare providers and medical insurers via a computer network.

In a **computer network,** each computer is like a house in your town, each having its own unique address called an *Internet protocol* (IP) address. A *router* is a networking device much like the post office because it routes information from the sending computer to the receiving computer.

When a patient's electronic medical record is sent to another computer, The Medical Manager program from the sending computer places the medical record into an **electronic envelope** called a *packet*. The packet is addressed with the address of the destination computer and the address of the computer sending the medical record. This information is **encrypted** to ensure the privacy of patients and adhere to HIPAA guidelines whether the company is using the Internet or personal intranet.

3. A Computer Program

When someone says she uses a computer to record, store, and retrieve a patient's medical records, she is really using a computer program to do these tasks. A computer program is a set of instructions that tell a computer what to do, when to do it, and how to do it.

There are many computer programs used in medical practices and hospitals. Some of these are familiar to you such as a word processor, spreadsheet, a browser to surf the Internet, and an e-mail program to send and receive e-mails.

Other computer programs are written specifically to manage a patient's medical and insurance records. Some of these are customized for a practice or hospital, while others are widely used throughout the medical industry.

A customized computer program electronically manages a patient's records the way the practice or hospital likes to manage patient records. The major disadvantages are technical support and training, which are expensive. The practice or hospital must hire a technical team to maintain the computer program and must train everyone to use it.

A computer program that is widely used in the medical industry may not manage patients' records in a way the practice or hospital likes. Two major advantages of using this computer program are that the firm that manufactures it provides technical support at a reasonable cost because it services many practices and hospitals. And since the computer program is widely used, the practice or hospital can usually hire employees who are already trained to use the computer program. One of the most popular patients' records manager computer program is The **Medical Manager** from the Emdeon Corporation. We'll give you some tips on how to use The Medical Manager to perform the most common medical insurance tasks later in this chapter.

4. Navigating a Computer Program

A computer program is started by double-clicking the computer program's icon on the computer display unless it's already preset to start up directly to a login window which then prompts you to enter your user ID and password.

The technician who administers the computer program assigns you a user ID and a temporary password when you join the practice or hospital. You'll be required to change the temporary password to a password that you create the first time you log on to the computer program. Only you know the new password. Should you forget it, the technician assigns you another temporary password, which you change the next time you log on. Periodically you'll be asked to change your password as a security measure.

Your **user ID** grants you the right to use certain features of the computer program required to do your job. You'll be electronically blocked from accessing features that are not within the scope of your responsibilities.

Your user ID and password are validated once you enter them into the computer program. A message is displayed if they are not validated. This usually occurs because either the user ID or password was mistyped. You'll be given another opportunity to log on. However, your user ID can be temporarily locked if you unsuccessfully try logging on several times in a row. This is a security precaution. If this happens to you, then simply contact the technician to unlock your user ID.

A main menu appears once you have successfully logged on. There are many styles, each displaying a list of features to choose from. Make your selection by entering the letter or number of the menu item or by clicking the menu item on the screen using your mouse depending on the style of menu used by the computer program.

A menu selection displays either another menu or a screen that contains a form similar to paper forms used in practices and hospitals that are not computerized. The cursor is automatically placed in the first item on the form. Anything you type is displayed at the cursor's position. You can move to other items on the form by using the tab key or by clicking the mouse on the item.

Some screens contain forms that display information, while others are used for entering new information or updating existing information. Still other forms are used to have the computer program search for and retrieve a patient's record.

The Medical Manager

A chapter on medical coding and billing software wouldn't be complete without a tour of the software itself. There are many medical coding and billing software applications in use today. A popular one is The Medical Manager.

The Medical Manager is designed for medium to large practices that handle hundreds of patients each day. Unfortunately, we don't have space in this book to show you every feature of The Medical Manager. However, we will walk you through four common routines that you'll perform as a medical insurance specialist. These are entering information about a new patient, recording the patient's encounter with a healthcare provider, posting a payment, and generating a patient statement.

5. New Patient Entry

When a new patient arrives, you must open a new guarantor account. A *guarantor* is the person who is financially responsible for medical costs. Enter information about the guarantor in the New Patient Entry screen, which is displayed by selecting New Patient from The Medical Manager's main menu.

The information that you will need to enter is self-explanatory and includes the guarantor's name and address and information about the guarantor's medical insurer. You'll also need to enter similar information about the guarantor's dependents who are covered by the policy. You'll see prompts at the bottom of the screen telling you the information that you need to enter into the screen.

First enter the guarantor's last name and then move on and enter other information on the form. The Medical Manager searches its electronic files to see if the name might already be on file. A list of names that match is displayed. Review each of them to determine if it is the same guarantor. No list appears if the name isn't found. You can search by account number, Social Security number, or ID, which is the policy number.

The Medical Manager automatically creates an account number and patient number. The account number identifies the guarantor, who is the holder of the medical insurance policy. The patient number identifies dependents who are covered under the policy. The patient number is divided into two parts by a decimal. To the left of the decimal is the account number, and to the right of the decimal is the patient's unique identifier. For example, Bob Smith is the guarantor and is assigned account number 10. His daughter Mary is assigned patient number 10.1.

HINT   *Click Help at the top of the screen if you find yourself lost. Press the Escape key to erase incorrect information on the form. Click the Exit button on the toolbar to start over at the New Patient Entry screen.*

You'll be asked to enter the number of insurance policies. Count only those insurance policies that cover the guarantor for services provided by the practice. Enter 0 if the guarantor doesn't have medical insurance.

You'll also be asked to enter the doctor number. This is the healthcare provider in the practice who has primary responsibility for the patient's care. Usually the doctor number is available from the office manager.

The Medical Manager can generate different kinds of walkout receipts and patient statements. A **walkout receipt** is the document given to the patient before leaving the office. The **patient statement** is a summary of the patient's account that is sent to the patient's home. You specify these with the bill type. The **bill type** is a two-part code. The first part identifies the walkout receipt, and the second part identifies the patient statement. For example, a bill type 11 means a walkout type 1 and a patient statement type 1. These are the default values. The office manager will decide which types to use for the practice.

The Consent field is used to indicate if the patient signed an authorization form and received a copy of the practice's privacy policy. Simply enter Y once the patient signs the form and receives the policy.

The Discount % field is the discount—if any—that the patient is to receive. Sometimes the practice discounts their fees for employees, relatives, and other healthcare professionals. The Medical Manager applies the discount when calculating fees.

The Budget Payment field is sometimes used if the patient has made a payment arrangement with the practice. It contains the amount of the regular payment.

Review all the information and then press F1 to process the form. All the information is lost if you exit before processing the information.

6. The Encounter

An **encounter** occurs when the patient is treated by the healthcare provider. This must be entered into The Medical Manager by selecting Procedure Entry from the main menu. The Medical Manager prompts you to enter the patient's account number or name, and then it displays the patient's account on the screen. Always review the account information to be sure you have the correct account.

A list of the patient's insurance plans is displayed. Select the insurer who has primary responsibility to cover the encounter. You'll also have the opportunity to enter secondary insurers.

Other information on the encounter screen is self-explanatory. One item is the doctor number of the healthcare provider who cared for the patient. In the case where the healthcare provider is a physician assistant, nurse practitioner, or another person other than the physician who provided care to the patient, the supervisor number field is used to enter the number of the physician who supervised the treatment.

Enter the procedure code and modifier, if needed; diagnosis and fee. Process the information before exiting the screen.

7. Posting Payment

When payments arrive, you must post them to the patient's account. As a medical billing specialist it is your responsibility that payments due are received timely and posted correctly. Any additional amount due must either be balanced or billed to the patient or their secondary insurance, if one is provided.

When payments are made by the insurer or the patient, they are entered into The Medical Manager where the payment is automatically deducted from the patient's outstanding balance. This is referred to as *posting the payment.* You can do this from the Procedure Entry screen or the Payment Entry screen, both of which are accessed through the main menu.

Use the Procedure Entry screen if the patient makes the payment. First enter the patient's account number to retrieve the account information. Make sure that the Primary Insurance # field is zero. This indicates that the patient—not the insurer—is making the payment.

The method of payment application field is used to identify how payment is being made. F is for full payment and P is the percentage of the Medicare-approved amount that the patient pays. If these don't apply, enter the percent of the payment that the patient is making. Then press F1 to process the payment.

The Payment Entry screen is used if payment is received by an insurer, but can also be used to post payments made by the patient. You get to the Payment Entry screen by selecting Payment Posting from the main menu. Once there you'll be asked to enter the patient's account number to display the patient's account information.

You'll have several posting options. These are Payment, Adjust, Transfer, Refund, and Void. Payment posts a payment to the patient's account. Adjust makes an adjustment to the account to correct any errors. Transfer moves a payment from one account to another if, for example, a payment was misposted. Refund is used to refund money to the patient or to an insurer. Void cancels the posting.

After selecting the type of posting, you enter the source of the payment. These are insurance or patient. When you choose insurance, you'll see a list of insurers who provide medical coverage for the patient. Select the insurer who is making the payment.

The Medical Manager automatically enters today's date as the reference date for the posting. You probably won't need to override it. Next, enter the voucher number (if one is provided) from the encounter form. The voucher number uniquely identifies the encounter. Enter whether payment is made by check, money (cash), or other and then enter the amount of the payment that you received.

8. Patient Statement

After payment is posted, the patient is issued a statement and lists encounters, charges, payments, and the patient's current balance. A statement is also issued periodically such as once a month if the patient has an outstanding balance.

You generate a statement from the Patient Statement screen, which is displayed by selecting the Billing and EDI from the main menu. You are given a choice between a trial and regular billing. A trial billing is a preliminary bill.

Next you are asked for a bill-thru date. A bill-thru date is the date of the last encounter that you want to appear on the bill. By default this is the current date, but sometimes you'll be asked to generate a statement for a different bill-thru date. For example, the patient may ask for a statement that reflects up to the end of last month. Therefore, the bill-thru date is the last day of the previous month.

Statements can be printed by account number, patient name, doctor, or zip code. These are referred to as *account order, patient name order, doctor order,* and *zip code order.* You'll be prompted to select an order.

Next, you'll be asked for the range of statements. The range can be one statement or several statements. Suppose you selected Account Order. You can enter one patient's account number or the account numbers for several patients depending on how many statements you want to print at the same time. The same applies for the other orders.

Next, you'll be asked to choose the scope of the billing statement. That is, do you want a particular type of bill or only delinquent statements? A *delinquent statement* is a statement for a patient whose payments have yet to be received in a timely manner.

Press F1 to process the statement, and you'll be asked if you want to use a previously designed format for the statement. If so, then choose the format. If not, then the default format is used for the statement. Press F1 and the statement is printed.

CASE STUDY

CASE 1
The practice manager of a large multi-practitioner practice has recently computerized the practice. She requires that their medical insurance specialist be familiar with computerization. During the interview, she asks you the following questions. What is the best response?

QUESTION 1. How can we connect our computers together to share patient and billing information?
ANSWER: Computers and computing devices, such as printers and disk drives, can be connected by using a computer network. Information is exchanged by computers and computing devices by using a router. A router is like an electronic post office that redirects information from the sending computer to the destination computer.

QUESTION 2. How can computerized patient information be protected?

ANSWER: To ensure compliance with HIPAA and provide privacy to patients, information that is stored and transmitted is encrypted. The sending computer encrypts the information and the destination computer is the only computer that deciphers the information.

QUESTION 3. Would we have to change the way we manage our patient records?

ANSWER: The computer application such as The Medical Manager may not manage patient records the same way as the practice manages them. There is a good chance that the practice will have to modify the way patient records are managed in order to take advantage of the efficiency of the computer application.

QUESTION 4. Why should we change our method of managing patient records since our method has worked well for decades?

ANSWER: The computer application offers a cost-effective way to store patient records and billing. Using popular computer applications, such as The Medical Manager, reduces training cost because medical insurance specialists are likely familiar with the application. Furthermore, the vendor who supplies that computer application ensures that the application is always compliant with regulatory requirements and provide 24/7 technical support to help the staff resolve problems related to the application.

FINAL CHECKUP

1. **The process of recording, storing, and retrieving information electronically is called**

    A. Forms processing

    B. Computerization

    C. Data searching

    D. All of the above

2. **A computer network is like**

    A. Your town

    B. A television

    C. A computer

    D. None of the above

3. **Telephone lines used in a network are like**

    A. Televisions

    B. Computers

    C. Streets in your town

    D. All of the above

4. **Each computer on a network is uniquely identified by an IP address.**

    A. True

    B. False

5. **A packet is an electronic envelope used to send patients' records electronically over a network.**

    A. True

    B. False

6. **An electronic envelope is carried over the network by**

    A. The network administrator

    B. Electricity or light waves

    C. The computer user

    D. All of the above

7. **Computer networks are connected together enabling a patient's medical record to be shared among hospitals.**

    A. True

    B. False

8. **A computer program is**

    A. A set of instructions that tell a computer what to do, when to do it, and how to do it.

    B. The cable that connects computers to the network.

    C. The cable that connects networks together.

    D. None of the above.

9. **Your user ID authorizes you to access features of the medical management software that are related to your job.**

    A. True

    B. False

10. **A temporary password must always be changed the first time that you successfully log on.**

    A. True

    B. False

CORRECT ANSWERS AND RATIONALES

1. B. Computerization.
2. A. Your town.
3. C. Streets in your town.
4. A. True.
5. A. True.
6. B. Electricity or light waves.
7. A. True.
8. A. A set of instructions that tell a computer what to do, when to do it, and how to do it.
9. A. True.
10. A. True.

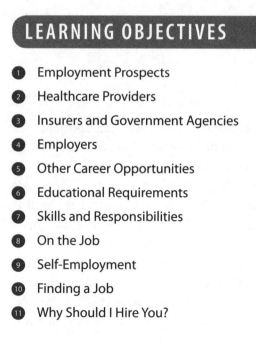

chapter 13

Finding Employment in the Healthcare Industry

LEARNING OBJECTIVES

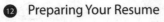 Preparing Your Resume

⑬ Designing Your Resume

⑭ Cover Letters

⑮ Online Submission

⑯ Job Search

⑰ You're in the Preliminary Finals

⑱ Preparing for the Interview

⑲ The Interview

⑳ After the Interview

KEY TERMS

American Association of Medical
  Assistants
American Health Information
  Management Association
Associate Degree
Business Smarts
Cash Flow
Certificate
Consultant

Cost
Educator
Entrepreneur
Finding Customers
Liability
Private Billing Practice
Profit
Writer

1. Employment Prospects

The time has arrived to find your first job as a medical insurance specialist. It's an exciting moment—and frightening too because you'll need to convince a prospective employer to bring you on board her healthcare team.

Finding a job is challenging, but not impossible since medical insurance specialists are in demand by healthcare providers in private practice, healthcare facilities, insurance companies, and private industry because they need someone to help them manage their medical benefits program.

Employment prospects for medical insurance specialists will remain favorable for the foreseeable future as the changing landscape of the insurance industry ensures a demand for professionals well versed in navigating the new requirements. The cost of healthcare further solidifying the need for medical insurance specialists, who are the professionals who ensure proper reimbursements are made in a timely fashion.

Medical insurance specialists are finding opportunities in many diverse areas of the economy including private healthcare practices, hospitals, same-day surgery centers, long-term care facilities, and third-party payers such as medical insurers and government agencies. Increasingly, medical insurance specialists are being sought by businesses in nearly every industry that need to find ways to ensure that their healthcare dollars are wisely spent.

2. Healthcare Providers

The way medical care is coded and billed has a direct financial impact on healthcare providers. Miscoding of a diagnosis or procedure can lead to an under-reimbursement resulting in the healthcare provider being underpaid for his services. This can have a serious ripple effect that might jeopardize the healthcare provider's financial survival if reimbursements fall below the cost of providing care to patients.

Improper coding and failure to provide necessary supporting documents delay reimbursements from insurers. This too financially impacts the healthcare provider because slow reimbursement means he must find other sources for money to pay the bills until he receives reimbursements from insurers.

Medical insurance specialists are trained to ensure that diagnoses and procedures are properly coded and all bills comply with requirements of medical insurers so that claims are expedited without delay.

3. Insurers and Government Agencies

Many people offset the cost of medical care by purchasing a medical insurance policy. The policy covers them for a range of medical conditions. The size of the range depends on the premium that the person can afford to pay. Insurers set the premium—and terms of the insurance policy—on certain assumptions based on experience.

The insurer needs to be sure that claims received on behalf of its client are covered by the client's insurance policy before the healthcare provider is reimbursed. Reimbursing for medical conditions that are outside of the terms of the insurance policy exposes the insurer to a financial loss since those medical conditions were not considered when the premium was set.

Some medical insurers control medical expenses by developing an ongoing financial relationship with healthcare providers where certain procedures are performed for a previously agreed upon rate.

Insurers employ medical insurance specialists to examine each claim to ensure that it falls within the patient's medical coverage. This also keeps the insurer financially sound.

4. Employers

Medical coverage is a desirable—but expensive—benefit for employees who join a company. Increasingly employers are looking for ways to lower their medical insurance cost while still maintaining a level of coverage that protects their employees from financial catastrophe should the employees fall ill.

Employers hold down healthcare costs by negotiating medical coverage with insurers. Negotiations involve fine-tuning the terms of a policy, terms that are unfamiliar to most employers. It is these details that, in some cases, determine the cost of the policy.

However, the medical insurance specialist is very familiar with these terms and is able to play a key role in advising an employer during negotiations with an insurer. Furthermore, the medical insurance specialist is the in-house advisor to make sure employees adhere to terms of their policy when receiving medical coverage.

5. Other Career Opportunities

There are employment opportunities for medical insurance specialists other than working directly for a healthcare provider or insurer. These include

- **Consultant.** A consultant advises a variety of clients on medical insurance issues such as attorneys, government agencies, employers, medical societies, and the media.
- **Educator.** A medical insurance specialist can join the full-time or part-time faculty of a college or a specialty school that trains future medical insurance specialists. He can also offer training to the healthcare provider's office staff.
- **Writer.** Medical insurers and others in the industry use talented medical insurance specialists to write brochures, newsletters, and booklets to explain medical insurance coverage in terms that the layperson can understand.
- **Entrepreneur.** An entrepreneur can offer a medical coding and billing service to healthcare providers who are unable to afford a staff medical insurance specialist.

- **Private billing practice.** A medical insurance specialist can provide a claims filing service to chronically ill patients, such as the elderly and disabled, who experience mounting medical bills to ensure that their medical costs are reimbursed.

6. Educational Requirements

Educational requirements vary. Although some medical insurance specialists learn their skills through on-the-job training or in-house training by their employer, many medical insurance specialists attend a formal training program. The training program usually includes courses in

- Medical terminology
- Anatomy and physiology
- Medical billing practices
- Medical coding practices
- Medical billing software applications

Some training programs also require that students complete courses in English composition, communications, and other general education courses.

Specialty schools and community colleges offer training. Some 4-year colleges also offer medical billing and coding training. Upon completing the program, students are awarded a certificate or an associate degree depending on the nature of the program and the institution offering it.

A certificate is usually obtained after completing a 1-year program consisting of courses directly related to medical billing and coding. An associate degree is obtained after a 2-year program that includes general education courses in addition to medical billing and coding courses.

A certificate or associate degree is sufficient education to fulfill the role of a medical insurance specialist. Many continue their education and obtain a 4-year degree in business or related area. This increases the opportunity of gaining additional responsibilities in an insurance company, healthcare facility, or directly from an employer.

7. Skills and Responsibilities

The **American Health Information Management Association** (AHIMA) and the **American Association of Medical Assistants** have defined the skills and responsibilities that are expected of the medical insurance specialist.

A medical insurance specialist should

- Work independently.
- Have high ethical standards.
- Pay attention to details.
- Have an understanding of anatomy and physiology.
- Know diagnosis and procedure coding.
- Be able to think critically.
- Communicate well.
- Understand medical terminology.
- Know how to enter data onto insurance claim forms.

The associations provide the medical insurance specialist's job description as follows:

- Review patient records and related documents.
- Properly code diagnoses, procedures, and services.
- Understand insurance rules and regulations.
- Operate office bookkeeping systems.
- Post charges and payments.
- Prepare and review claims for accuracy.
- Review insurance payments.
- Appeal claims when necessary.
- Update staff about new regulations.
- Explain to patients how their insurance affects their healthcare.

8. On the Job

Employers use the job description defined by the AHIMA and the American Association of Medical Assistants as a guide to create their own job description for a medical insurance specialist. The job that you perform is likely to differ from the suggested job description.

Here are tasks that you are expected to perform in nearly all positions:

- Keep up-to-date on rules and regulations governing claims for insurers.
- Submit claims and invoice patients.
- Post charges to patients' accounts.

- Post payments and reimbursement to patients' accounts.
- Report on the status of claims and forecast reimbursements to help with the cash flow analysis for the practice.
- Process responses from insurers.
- Appeal claims that are denied or underpaid.
- Keep staff informed of insurance regulations and laws.
- Make sure pretreatment authorizations are requested and received.
- Explain the claims process to patients.

9. Self-Employment

While many dream of becoming their own boss so that they can control their own destiny, being your own boss isn't without risks that are not experienced by employees. Consider these factors before starting your own medical billing and coding practice.

- **Finding customers.** Most healthcare providers have a need for someone to handle their medical billing and coding, but that need is usually already filled. Therefore, you'll have to convince healthcare providers that you offer a better value than their present arrangement for submitting claims. This is especially difficult to do if you are just starting out in the business because the healthcare provider has to put his financial well-being into the hands of someone who may not have a proven track record.

- **Finding enough customers.** Private medical billing and coding practices are able to offer services at a reasonable cost because their expenses are shared among many clients. One customer probably won't support your practice because it is cheaper to hire a medical insurance specialist than to pay your fee. Expect to finance your practice yourself without depending on fees until you've built it up.

- **Liability.** Consult an attorney to determine your liability should problems arise. As a vendor to the healthcare provider, you have greater liability than you would have as an employee. For example, miscoding a claim can get you fired as an employee. Miscoding a claim can get you sued as a vendor because the healthcare provider loses money because of your mistake. Many things can go wrong and result in litigation.

- **Cost.** Carefully itemize the expenses involved in running your practice. These include rent, utilities, computers, liability insurance, medical insurance, advertising and marketing, accounting services, and many other expenses. And this list grows once you hire employees. It is best to consult an accountant who already has a medical billing and coding practice as a client so you don't overlook any expenses.

- **Profit.** Profit is money left after expenses. It is not fees you receive from healthcare providers. A common misconception is that fees are equivalent to the salary you will receive as an employee. Your salary is equivalent to profit.

- **Cash flow.** Cash flow is the accounting term that describes when you receive money and when you spend money. In the ideal practice, you receive money in time to pay your bills; otherwise you'll need to dip into your savings or borrow cash to pay them. You receive money on your scheduled payday as an employee. However, you receive your fee whenever the healthcare provider gets around to paying you as a vendor. Some healthcare providers are prompt payers and others don't pay for months.

- **Business smarts.** Do you have the know-how to operate a business? Speak with an accountant and your attorney about what it takes to be an entrepreneur. If possible, discuss your plans with someone who already operates a medical billing and coding practice.

Consider acquiring one or more certifications that are awarded by professional organizations. These certify that you passed a standardized competency test in medical billing and coding. Here are popular certifications.

- The National Electronic Billers Alliance (NEBA)
  - Certified Healthcare Reimbursement Specialist (CHRS)
- The American Academy of Professional Coders (AAPC)
  - Certified Professional Coder Apprentice (CPC-A)
  - Certified Professional Coder–Hospital Apprentice (CPC-HA)
  - Certified Professional Coder (CPC)
  - Certified Professional Coder–Hospital
- The AHIMA
  - Certified Coding Associate (CCA)
  - Certified Coding Specialist (CCS)
  - Certified Coding Specialist–Physician-Based (CCS-P)
- The American Medical Billing Association (AMBA)
  - Certified Medical Reimbursement Specialist (CMRS)

10. Finding a Job

Finding a new position as a medical insurance specialist requires careful preparation and devising a strategy to sell a prospective employer that you will be a valued member of her healthcare team. Begin by telling yourself that you are a medical insurance specialist who can handle any situation that might arise. You have to believe in yourself before you can convince others to believe in you.

Once you make your first sale—to yourself—then you'll start to develop the right mindset to project a winning attitude to a potential employer. A winning attitude demonstrates that you

- Can take direction.
- Strive for excellence.
- Contribute to the healthcare provider's goal of caring for patients while earning a profit.
- Are responsible for your actions.
- Can solve your own problems.

Next, set realistic expectations about finding a new position. In the ideal world, you simply walk into a healthcare provider's office, present your credentials, and start work. This rarely happens. Finding the right fit can take months of sending out resumes and going on interviews.

You'll be rejected more times than you'll be offered employment. Learn from these rejections. Ask yourself—and possibly the person who interviewed you—why someone else was chosen. If you ask your prospective employer this, be sure to ask in a positive way. Say, "Thank you for considering me. I enjoyed our conversation. I'm always looking for ways to improve. Would you mind sharing with me why you didn't feel I was right for the position?" Sometimes the response will surprise you.

Above all, keep a positive attitude and don't become discouraged because there is a position for nearly everyone; you simply haven't found it yet.

11. Why Should I Hire You?

A prospective employer looks for someone

- Whose personality, work habits, and attitude complement that of other members of the healthcare team.
- Who can contribute to making money or saving money for the practice.

Take a piece of paper and write down evidence that you meet these qualifications. Evidence includes your previous experience and training. For example, you might note that you learned techniques on how to avoid reimbursement delays during your training as a medical insurance specialist. This increases cash flow and thereby saves money by reducing the need to borrow funds while awaiting reimbursement.

If this isn't your first medical insurance specialist position, then you might say how you were a team player at your present employer and share experiences that demonstrate your ability to process claims.

If this is your first medical insurance specialist position, then note how your current skills are transferable to the medical insurance specialist position. You could say that in your present position you place orders with vendors, manage purchase orders, and ensure that the right goods or services are received. These tasks correspond somewhat to preparing claims and verifying that reimbursements are received.

Think of experiences that illustrate how you worked independently and under pressure because these will be important selling points to include in your resume. Be honest because you'll be using this information to build your resume, which will be verified by your prospective employer.

12. Preparing Your Resume

A resume is your sales brochure that describes your accomplishments and how an employer can leverage those accomplishments to make money or save money. Your resume, as with any sales brochure, is designed to make an employer aware of you and encourage the employer to take a closer look at you. That's all. It opens the door to a job, but it doesn't get you hired.

As you prepare your resume, keep in mind that a prospective employer might receive nearly 100 resumes—sometimes hundreds of resumes depending on the position. The employer will probably whittle down the pile to 10 resumes that catch his eye. Your job is to write an eye-catching resume that places you in the 10 he picks.

This doesn't mean using pretty pictures, dramatic colors, and other clever ways advertisers try to get your attention in a sales brochure. Using these techniques in a resume usually shows that you don't know how to prepare a professional resume.

Eye catching means that at the beginning of your resume you clearly match your qualifications to the job description published by the employer. This eliminates the need for the employer to search through your resume looking for experience that might meet the qualifications for the position.

Let's say that the employer says the ideal candidate for the position should have

1. Certification as a medical insurance specialist or equivalent experience.
2. Experience with a geriatric practice.
3. Be an expert on Medicare and Medicaid.

At the beginning of your resume you should write

1. Certified as a medical insurance specialist by Bergen Community College.
2. Five years as a medical insurance specialist for a three-physician geriatric practice.
3. Five years preparing Medicare and Medicaid claims.

Notice that each job requirement is matched with an experience. Also notice that we try to use as many of the words from the job description as possible in our experience. This is important because sometimes an assistant is given the job description and told to select resumes that match it. Using the same words makes the comparison easy. Large employers use a computer to sift through resumes looking for keywords such as those used in the job description.

13. Designing Your Resume

Design your resume from the viewpoint of the reader. Ask yourself, "What is the most important information the reader needs to know?" And then make sure that information is clearly the first piece of information on your resume.

Remember that the employer is sorting 100 resumes looking for 10 or as few as 3 prospects who he'll meet in person. Therefore, he might spend less than 15 seconds answering the question, "Does the person's background match the job description?"

There are many designs to choose from for your resume. Each has its advantages and disadvantages. We'll use a design that organizes your resume into four sections, placing the information the employer needs to know up front. These are

- **Contact information.** The first section is at the top of the page and consists of your name, address, phone number, and e-mail address. Be sure to use your personal e-mail address and not your employer's e-mail address. If possible, have an answering machine attached to the telephone so you won't miss a call inviting you in for an interview.
- **Highlights.** The second section contains highlights of your experience. This section is the most important because it is where you match your

experience to each item in the job description. List these items in the same order in which they appear in the job description. Keep each item brief. Give just enough information to show that you have what the employer is looking for. No more than a sentence. Think of this as a headline in a newspaper. A newspaper headline contains keywords—no details—that encourage you to read more about the story.

- **Experience.** The third section is where you list your experience in reverse chronological order placing your current or most recent position first. Only go back 10 years. Each item should have a heading that includes your title, employer's name and address, and the start and end date of your employment. Write a brief paragraph or a bulleted list below the heading that summarizes your job. Each item in the highlights section must have a corresponding item in the experience section where you elaborate on your experience. Think of an item in the highlights section as a headline and an item in the experience section as the story. It is important that you use the same words in the item in the paragraph as you used in the item in the highlights section in order to link both items.

- **Education.** The fourth section contains your education in chronological order. List the institution, years attended, and certificate or degree received. Leave the certificate or degree blank if you didn't complete the program. Include in-house training and seminars that are relevant to the position.

Writing Your Resume

Limit your resume to one page—two pages is the maximum—because the employer isn't likely to read beyond the top half of the first page. By that time the employer should already know if you are a candidate for the position.

Be sure to have someone who is a good editor to proofread your resume. Don't rely on your word processor's spelling and grammar checker. Your misspelled word might actually be a word in the spell checker's dictionary.

Just the Facts

Describe your experience accurately. You can exaggerate, but you shouldn't mislead because your prospective employer will conduct a background check and discover inconsistencies in your resume. An employer is likely to overlook exaggerations if your resume isn't misleading.

Also be aware that some employers hire you before completing the background check. This means that you might be working for your new employer for a couple of months while she verifies information on your resume. Anything misleading could be a cause to terminate your employment.

For example, don't say that you are in a medical insurance specialist certification program if you haven't as yet been officially accepted into the program. Likewise, it is misleading if you say that you handled medical coding and billing for a healthcare provider when in reality you were a medical receptionist who assisted the healthcare provider's medical insurance specialist with coding and billing.

In these situations you could say that in conjunction with your responsibilities as a medical receptionist, you assisted the staff medical insurance specialist in coding and billing claims. You applied for the evening certification program at Bergen Community College and expect to begin training in 2 months.

Making Your Resume a Work of Art

Make your resume look presentable by

- Using 1-in margins around the page.
- Capitalizing the first character of each word in a heading.
- Making headings bold.
- Single spacing between lines.
- Double spacing between sections.
- Using bulleted lists inside of paragraphs where possible to make your points pop out.
- Using 8 × 11 in, 16- to 25-pound high-quality bond paper.
- Using a matching envelope when possible.
- Printing the address on the envelope using your computer. Don't handwrite it and don't use a label. Handwriting is unprofessional and a label makes it seem like junk mail.

Filling in the Holes

Once you have finished writing the draft of your resume, read it as if you were a prospective employer. Look at the job requirements and compare them to your resume. Within 10 seconds can you tell if you meet those requirements by reading your resume? If so, then your resume accomplished its mission. If not, then you'll need to polish the wording of your resume.

Look for inconsistencies and things that don't make sense. If you say in the highlights section that you handled medical coding and billing for 5 years, then this experience should be apparent in your experience section. If it isn't clear, then your prospective employer might question the accuracy of the information on your resume.

Clarify any gaps in your work experience. A prospective employer wants to know what you've been doing for the past 5 or 10 years, so he'll expect to find a chronological path in the experience and the education sections of your resume.

Ideally you'll have a consistent work record where you've stayed with an employer for at least a couple of years before changing to another employer. Employers will understand if you were laid off from a position and took a few months to find a new one if you explain this in the experience section of your resume.

However, some inconsistencies signal a red flag possibly disqualifying you as a candidate. For example, a pattern where you stay with an employer for less than 2 years indicates instability and is likely to eliminate you from contention before you have an opportunity to explain yourself.

Another red flag is whether you consistently change the nature of your employment. Ideally you've stayed within the medical insurance or healthcare industry for your career. Employers understand if your experience is in another industry and are changing careers by switching to the healthcare industry. However, you might be disqualified from consideration if there is a pattern of changing industries frequently.

Target Your Resume

A common error when searching for a job is to send a prospective employer a resume that isn't targeted for the open position. In doing this, you leave it up to the employer to match your experience to the job description, which is risky because she probably doesn't have time to do it.

Customizing a resume for each position that you apply for might seem like a burden, but it isn't if you follow a few simple steps:

- Use a word processor to write a general resume. A general resume includes sections that change very little. These are the contact information section, the experience section, and the education section.
- Save the resume to your computer disk.
- Open the general resume each time you want to apply for a position.
- Insert the highlights section, which provides an item-by-item comparison of your experience to the job description.
- If necessary, modify each item in the experience section to focus on requirements of the job description.
- Save the resume in a different file on your computer disk.

14. Cover Letters

A cover letter is a one-page letter that asks a prospective employer to consider you for an open position and is accompanied by your resume. Both should be on the same size and type of paper and be sent in a business-size envelope. Don't staple the cover letter to the resume.

The objective of a cover letter is to have the prospective employer read your resume. And to do this you must think like a salesperson who tells just enough about a product to grab the customer's attention.

There are seven sections of a cover letter:

1. **Return name and address.** It is best to use your word processor to create a letterhead where your name, address, and contact information is in relatively large, bold type at the top of the cover letter. You can be creative in your design as long as it stays within acceptable letterhead style.

2. **Addressee.** This contains the prospective employer's name and address. Be sure to include the full proper name, title, company name, and address. Place this along the left margin of the letter.

3. **Salutation.** Begin by using *Dear* followed by *Mr., Ms, Miss, Mrs.,* or *Dr.* and the person's formal name. Always address a prospective employer formally until you become on a first-name basis with him.

4. **Opening sentence.** The opening sentence is where you introduce yourself and tell the prospective employer why you sent the cover letter.

5. **The sales pitch.** This section contains a paragraph that gives the prospective employer reasons for reading your resume. These reasons are contained in the highlights section of your resume. You simply summarize the highlights in this paragraph.

6. **Closing sentence.** This sentence gives the prospective employer direction, such as "I'll give you a call in a few days so we can discuss your position in detail."

7. **Signature.** The last section contains your signature. Make sure that you type your full name and leave room so you can sign the cover letter.

15. Online Submission

Many large employers require job applicants to apply over the Internet on their Web site by clicking the link to their online application and then filling in information that is normally required for an application.

Alternatively, you might be permitted to send a cover letter and your resume instead of filling in the application. Your cover letter and resume must be in an electronic file, which it usually already is if you created it using a word processor. Follow the steps on the Web site, and a copy of your cover letter and resume files will be sent over the Internet to the prospective employer's computer where it is placed into a database.

Someone in human resources then queries the database for resumes that seem to meet the criteria for the position. This means there is a chance that a person won't review your resume unless the computer deems you qualified.

When a position is open, the human resources department enters the job description and search criteria into its computer. The search criteria specify the conditions that must be met for the computer to forward a resume to a human resource representative.

There are two ways to increase the chances of the computer picking your resume.

- Use in your resume as many words as possible that are contained in the job description. Spell out and use abbreviations. The computer likely compares words in the job description with the resume.

- Save your file as plain text rather than as a Word document. Plain text excludes formatting, which may interfere with picking your resume.

16. Job Search

With preparations completed, you're ready to begin looking for a job. Begin your job search by visiting your school's placement office. Frequently, prospective employers contact the placement office to fill open positions because the school's staff can filter unqualified candidates. Also former students who have moved into management look to help current students find employment.

Keep in mind that many schools encourage former graduates to continue to use the placement office as a source for employment opportunities for years after they graduate. Some schools hold open houses where prospective employers, students, and former students can meet and explore career opportunities.

Probably the most common way to find a job is by word of mouth. Employers tend to place candidates at the top of the line if a current employee recommends them. Ask friends and relatives if they know of someone who works for a medical insurer, healthcare facility, or a healthcare provider who can help you find a position.

Employer Web sites are also a very good source for open positions. Make a list of all the possible employers in your area, visit their Web site each week, and look at their open positions and then apply online.

Find the name and e-mail address of the person who is responsible for medical billing and coding for each prospective employer on your list. You can find the information on the employer's Web site or give the employer a call. Send an e-mail telling the person of your desire to join that department sometime in the future and ask for advice on how to accomplish your goal.

Visit one of the many online employment Web sites such as monster.com and search for open positions in your area.

17. You're in the Preliminary Finals

You'll receive a call if the prospective employer feels your resume matches the job description asking you to come in for an interview. Be accommodating and schedule the interview for a time that is convenient to both of you.

Keep your conversation brief. Focus on arranging the interview and not on your qualifications or on the position. Leave that for the interview.

Make sure to obtain

- The date and time.
- The name of the person you will be meeting.
- The spelling of the person's name and title.
- Directions to the building.
- Instructions for parking.
- Instructions for meeting the person. Sometimes you'll be asked to wait in the reception area.

18. Preparing for the Interview

You have one chance to make a good first impression, so you'll need to prepare yourself for the interview. The prospective employer is looking for you to prove two things during the interview—you fit in the team and you have the skills to do the job.

Here are things to do to prepare for your interview.

- Visit the organization's Web site and learn about the organization and its goals.

- Study the job description and be prepared to explicitly describe how your background meets the job requirements.

- Update yourself on the latest medical billing and coding trends so that you can discuss them during the interview.

- Refresh your memory on some unique requirements imposed by major insurers. You'll then be prepared to mention these to show your depth of knowledge in the field.

- Review your resume for inconsistencies that might raise doubts over your qualifications—and then prepare a rationale to explain them.

- Dress to impress. Get your hair trimmed and shoes shined, and wear clothes that fit well and are clean.

- Bring three copies of you resume.

- Get a good night's sleep before the interview.

- Drive by the employer's location a day or so before the interview if you are not familiar with it.

- Prepare alternative routes in case traffic is backed up on the day of the interview.

19. The Interview

This is the moment that you've been waiting for. It is time to give your sales pitch and convince the prospective employer that you're the right person for the job. Get up early on the day of the interview. Listen to the traffic report so you know which route to take to the interview. Plan to arrive in the vicinity 30 minutes before the interview. This gives you time to find the place. Enter the building 15 minutes before the interview. This gives you time for a bathroom stop.

Consider yourself a guest, but try to be natural and friendly as if you are already a part of the team and confident that you can do the job. The interviewer will start by asking an open-ended question about your background such as about your school and previous employers. Respond by saying these were positive experiences. Don't speak negatively about them.

If you answered these questions satisfactorily, the interviewer will begin describing the position to you. At this point, many interviewers have decided that you are a good candidate for the position. The clue that you're a finalist is when the interviewer talks about salary. They usually don't reach this topic unless they think you are a very good fit for the job.

Here are a few tips to get you through the interview.

- Project a positive attitude when greeting the interviewer.
- Start with some small talk, such as about the weather or traffic conditions, while walking to the site of the interview.
- Let the interviewer begin the conversation once you settle in.
- Be a good listener and don't interrupt the interviewer when she's speaking.
- Respond to questions clearly and in complete sentences.
- Think before you speak. Avoid thinking out loud. You are being judged on everything you say and the way you say it.
- Sit up straight and maintain eye contact with the interviewer at all times.
- Keep responses to the point but friendly.
- Ask the interviewer to clarify any questions that you don't fully understand.
- Be honest and say you don't know the answer rather than trying to bluff the interviewer.
- Ask your own questions. Find out why the position is open. You might learn there has been a high turnover in that position. If so, then you might want to pass up this opportunity because the employer is quick to terminate employees.
- Use correct terminology when responding to questions or asking questions.

End the interview on a positive note. Ask the interviewer when she is planning to reach a decision. Find out how many candidates are in the current round of interviews. Are there any in-house candidates? Employers tend to hire within before going outside the organization. Determine if there will be further interviews. Sometimes the interviewer is the first of several people who approve a new hirer.

A good interviewer will leave you with the impression that you are the lead candidate for the position when in reality he might have already hired someone before you entered his office. So don't read too much into the interview until you are invited back for a follow-up interview or are offered a job.

20. After the Interview

Follow up the interview with an e-mail to everyone who interviewed you thanking them for spending time with you. Include in the letter the one reason why they should offer you the position.

Consider sending a letter rather than an e-mail. A letter is likely to get more attention than an e-mail because not many people send letters, but some interviewers can receive nearly 100 e-mails a day. The letter should be on the same paper that you used for your resume.

Make note of the date of the interview and the date that the interviewer expects to reach a decision on the position. Send an e-mail to the interviewer a week to 10 days following the interview telling her that you are interested in pursuing the position and ask for the status of your application.

You'll receive a call if the employer intends to offer you the position. It is during this call when the employer will finalize the terms of employment such as work hours, vacation, benefits, and salary. Once terms are settled, you'll receive the official offer in the mail.

However, you might receive a call, an e-mail, or a letter telling you that the position was offered to another person. Remain professional and polite. Although you didn't get the position, you made important contacts that might help you obtain a position in the future within their organization. Send a thank you e-mail or letter and then plan to send follow-up e-mails or letters twice a year or every quarter reminding them that you're still interested in joining their organization.

CASE STUDY

CASE 1

You applied for a medical insurance specialist position working for a large practitioner's office. A week after submitting your resume, you receive a call for an interview with the office manager and with three of the principal practitioners of the practice. You are asked the following questions. What is the best response?

QUESTION 1. Why should we hire you?
ANSWER: I want to contribute to the group practice goal of caring for patients while earning a profit by ensuring that the group practice receives the maximum allowable reimbursements.

QUESTION 2. How can you ensure that maximum allowable reimbursements are received?
ANSWER: I keep up-to-date on rules and regulations that govern claims for insurers and incorporate those rules and regulations into standardized medical coding and billing practices for the practice group.

QUESTION 3. What makes you stand out from other candidates for this position?
ANSWER: I work independently, pay attention to detail, able to think critically, and I know diagnosis and procedure coding and able to successfully interact with insurers, practitioners, staff, and patients.

QUESTION 4. Name one procedure that you implemented to help a practice group?
ANSWER: I report on the status of claims and forecast reimbursements to help the practice group develop effective cash flow analysis for the practice.

FINAL CHECKUP

1. **Employment prospects for medical insurance specialists will remain favorable because**

   A. Medical billing is becoming less important to the healthcare industry.
   B. Medical billing is automated.
   C. The changing landscape of the insurance industry ensures a demand for professionals well versed in navigating the new requirements.
   D. Automation has eliminated all errors.

2. **Insurers need medical insurance specialists because**

   A. Of regulatory requirements.
   B. The insurer needs to be sure that claims received on behalf of his client are covered by the client's insurance policy before the healthcare provider is reimbursed.
   C. Health insurers are incurring severe financial losses.
   D. Health insurers can no longer hire nurses to manage medical claims.

3. **Private billing practices focus on**

   A. Elderly and disabled who experience mounting medical bills.
   B. Only private practitioners.
   C. Small physician practitioners and the nurse practitioner market.
   D. Major healthcare facilities.

4. **Many medical insurance specialists attend a formal training program.**

   A. True
   B. False

5. **Miscoding a claim can get you sued as a vendor because the healthcare provider loses money because of your mistake.**

   A. True
   B. False

6. Cash flow is the accounting term that describes
   A. When you receive reimbursement.
   B. When you submit a claim.
   C. When you pay bills.
   D. When you receive money and when you spend money.

7. A resume is your sales brochure that describes your accomplishments and how an employer can leverage those accomplishments to make money or save money.
   A. True
   B. False

8. What should you be able to do within 10 seconds of reading your resume?
   A. Tell if you are reliable.
   B. Tell if you are certified.
   C. Tell if you meet the job requirements.
   D. Tell if you are competent.

9. You should target your resume to a specific employment opportunity.
   A. True
   B. False

10. You should never submit your resume over the Internet.
    A. True
    B. False

CORRECT ANSWERS AND RATIONALES

1. C. The changing landscape of the insurance industry ensures a demand for professionals well versed in navigating the new requirements.
2. B. The insurer needs to be sure that claims received on behalf of his client are covered by the client's insurance policy before the healthcare provider is reimbursed.
3. A. Elderly and disabled who experience mounting medical bills.
4. A. True.
5. A. True.
6. D. When you receive money and when you spend money.
7. A. True.
8. C. Tell if you meet the job requirements.
9. A. True.
10. A. False.

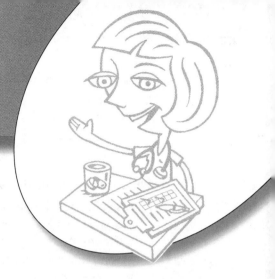

Final Exam

1. **What is an electroencephalogram?**

    A. Diagram of tissue electrical activity.

    B. Recording of tissue electrical activity.

    C. Recording of the brain's electrical activity.

    D. None of the above.

2. **What does an insured pay to the insurer for healthcare coverage?**

    A. A down payment

    B. A reimbursement

    C. A premium

    D. None of the above

3. **What is a healthcare encounter?**

    A. An encounter is whenever the patient calls the practitioner's office.

    B. An encounter is whenever the patient engages the practitioner for service.

    C. An encounter is whenever the patient pays a co-pay.

    D. An encounter is whenever the patient's insurer pays a reimbursement.

4. **Emdeon or Passport are systems used to assist patient pay co-payments.**

    A. True

    B. False

5. **A claim that does not adhere to policies of the insurer is called**

   A. Compliance
   B. Bounding
   C. Noncompliance
   D. Fraud

6. **What is the reconciliation process?**

   A. Assignment of the claim control number.
   B. The process of matching a claim on the remittance advice with claims submitted to the insurer.
   C. Making sure the claim control number hasn't been already used.
   D. Resolving differences among practitioner and patient.

7. **What does a patient tell a practitioner during a visit?**

   A. Signs
   B. Symptoms
   C. Signs and symptoms
   D. Treatment plans

8. **Insurers need medical insurance specialists because**

   A. Of regulatory requirements.
   B. The insurer needs to be sure that claims received on behalf of his client are covered by the client's insurance policy before the healthcare provider is reimbursed.
   C. Health insurers are incurring severe financial losses.
   D. Health insurers can no longer hire nurses to manage medical claims.

9. **Hemorrhoidectomy is removal of a hernia.**

   A. True
   B. False

10. **When you determine a call is an emergency, ask**

    A. What is the nature of the emergency?
    B. What is the address of the emergency?
    C. What is the caller's telephone number?
    D. All of the above.

11. **Consideration in a contract is**

    A. Money
    B. Performance of an action
    C. A house
    D. All of the above

12. **Qualifications to receive Medicaid are uniform throughout the United States.**
    A. True
    B. False

13. **An average person who fails to exercise ordinary care commits**
    A. Malpractice
    B. Negligence
    C. Feasence
    D. All of the above

14. **The scheduling method that gives the same appointment to two or more patients is called**
    A. Computer scheduling
    B. Double booking
    C. Wave scheduling
    D. None of the above

15. **How does an insurer spread the risk of high reimbursements?**
    A. Insuring a group of people
    B. Insuring individuals
    C. Insuring only groups of young people
    D. All of the above

16. **If the patient has two jobs and each employer provides health insurance, which policy is the primary policy?**
    A. The policy that is in effect the longest is the primary policy.
    B. The policy that is in effect the shortest is the primary policy.
    C. Either policy can be considered the primary policy.
    D. The patient selects which of the policies is the primary policy.

17. **Errors in medical coding and billing also affect patient relations because**
    A. All charges rejected by the insurer are paid by the patient.
    B. The patient may be charged amounts not reimbursed by the insurer as a result of medical billing and coding errors.
    C. The insurer may be charged amounts not reimbursed by the patient as a result of medical billing and coding errors.
    D. The patient may refuse to pay anything except the co-pay.

18. **What are nonpars?**
    A. Healthcare providers who participate in the payer's program.
    B. Healthcare providers who do not participate in the payer's program.
    C. The appeals process.
    D. Claim examiner.

19. **What are a patient's physiological reserves?**

    A. A form of co-pay.

    B. Medication that is prescribed by the practitioner.

    C. A comprehensive health insurance policy.

    D. The capabilities of the body to repair itself.

20. **Private billing practices focus on**

    A. Elderly and disabled who experience mounting medical bills.

    B. Only private practitioners.

    C. Small physician practitioners and the nurse practitioner market.

    D. Major healthcare facilities.

21. **Medical insurers earn a profit by**

    A. Investing premiums.

    B. Denying claims.

    C. Extending the time between when the claim is filed and the claim is paid.

    D. All of the above.

22. **What is hepatitis?**

    A. Liver inflammation

    B. Hip inflammation

    C. Liver spots on the eyelids

    D. None of the above

23. **A practitioner's assistant is**

    A. Licensed to perform some of a practitioner's duties under the direct supervision of a practitioner.

    B. A phlebotomist.

    C. Responsible in the medical office.

    D. All of the above.

24. **An exclusion is an event covered by the insurance policy.**

    A. True

    B. False

25. **What happens when a claim is approved by the insurer?**

    A. Once the claim is approved for payment, the medical billing and coding professional sends the insurer a remittance advice (RA) that details all the procedures that were listed on the claim and the reimbursement for each of them.

    B. Once the claim is approved for payment, the patient sends the insurer a remittance advice (RA) that details all the procedures that were listed on the claim and the reimbursement for each of them.

C. Once the claim is approved for payment, the healthcare provider sends a remittance advice (RA) that details all the procedures that were listed on the claim and the reimbursement for each of them.

D. Once verified, the claim is approved for payment and the healthcare provider is sent a remittance advice (RA) that details all the procedures that were listed on the claim and the reimbursement for each of them.

26. **Itemizing fees may be considered**

A. Mismatch coding

B. Reconstruction of documentation

C. Omissions

D. Double billing

27. **An F response code means that the claim is approved.**

A. True

B. False

28. **Practitioners must be licensed by the Food & Drug Administration to prescribe medications.**

A. True

B. False

29. **Any items that appear more than once in a claim may be considered double billing.**

A. True

B. False

30. **Patient information entered incorrectly into the healthcare facility's records can delay reimbursements.**

A. True

A. False

31. **How does a person determine whether the healthcare insurance is worth the premium?**

A. You first must estimate your healthcare expenses of your current illness.

B. You first must estimate your healthcare expenses without medical coverage.

C. You first must estimate your healthcare expenses of all your previous illness.

D. You first must estimate your premium cost for all your previous illness.

32. **With fixed office hours, patients do not require an appointment to see the practitioner.**

A. True

B. False

33. **Endocarditis in an infection of the outer part of the heart.**

    A. True

    B. False

34. **Which of the following is inflammation of the gums?**

    A. Gingivitis

    B. Gingivosis

    C. Gingia

    D. Gingivectomy

35. **Office hours are scheduled to reduce waiting times for patients and make the best use of the healthcare team's time.**

    A. True

    B. False

36. **The member of the healthcare team who is responsible for maintaining, storing, and retrieving patient records is the**

    A. Phlebotomist

    B. Medical technician

    C. Medical records specialist

    D. None of the above

37. **How can you verify that a patient's health insurance is active?**

    A. Ask the patient.

    B. Ask the patient to show the health insurance ID card.

    C. Use the medical insurer's Web site, by telephone, or through an insurance eligibility verification system.

    D. Ask the practitioner.

38. **Mismatch coding occurs when an element of the claim is not consistent with other elements, such as the gender is coded as male for a diagnosis of a hysterectomy.**

    A. True

    B. False

39. **CDA messaging is used to share a portion of a patient's healthcare record with another healthcare facility.**

    A. True

    B. False

40. **You should never submit your resume over the Internet.**

    A. True

    B. False

41. Claims that pass the edit enter the medical review stage of the claims adjudication process that is performed by the payer's medical review department.

    A. True
    B. False

42. An investigator reviewing a claim may not examine other claims to determine if a pattern of fraud exists.

    A. True
    B. False

43. What is electronic funds transfer?

    A. The system used to appeal reimbursement claims.
    B. The system used to submit reimbursement claims.
    C. Transfer of reimbursements directly into the healthcare provider's bank account.
    D. The system used by insurers to assess reimbursement claims.

44. If the patient is a child who lives with both parents and is covered by two medical policies—provided by each parent's employer—primary coverage is provided by the employer of the parent whose birthday comes second in the calendar year.

    A. True
    B. False

45. For an insured covered by an HMO, except for emergencies, the insured must use healthcare providers and healthcare facilities that are part of the HMO. Care received outside the HMO that is not approved by the primary care practitioner isn't reimbursed.

    A. True
    B. False

46. A PET scan is a(n)

    A. Computerized image of the metabolic activity of body tissues.
    B. Magnetic resonance imaging (MRI) to measure activity at the cellular level.
    C. X-ray of the hepatic and common bile ducts.
    D. None of the above.

47. Medicaid is a joint program operated by the federal and state governments to provide medical insurance for the indigent.

    A. True
    B. False

48. A splenectomy is removal of the spleen.

    A. True
    B. False

49. An exclusive provider organization is a network of healthcare providers who have contracts with specific health insurers. Policyholders are required to select a primary-care practitioner who is a member of the EPO. The primary-care practitioner provides preventative care and primary care, and refers the policyholder to a specialist when necessary.

    A. True
    B. False

50. Unbundling occurs when a claim contains separate procedures that should have been grouped into a bundled procedure.

    A. True
    B. False

51. What is the role of The Joint Commission?

    A. The Joint Commission accredits hospitals and establishes standards for healthcare facilities.
    B. The Joint Commission accredits medical schools.
    C. The Joint Commission oversees physician license exams.
    D. The Joint Commission certifies physician specialties.

52. A resume is your sales brochure that describes your accomplishments and how an employer can leverage those accomplishments to make money or save money.

    A. True
    B. False

53. An explanation of benefit is

    A. Sent by the insurer to the patient when the claim is adjudicated.
    B. Sent by the practitioner to the patient when the claim is adjudicated.
    C. Sent by the insurer to the patient when the claim is denied.
    D. Sent by the insurer to the practitioner when the claim is denied.

54. A deductible is the amount that the patient will have to pay before the medical insurance will pay a reimbursement.

    A. True
    B. False

55. Has a lifetime payout provision be eliminated from healthcare insurance?

    A. Yes, by the Affordable Care Act.
    B. No, the Affordable Care Act prohibits exclusion of a lifetime payout clause.
    C. Yes, however, lifetime limits can apply to healthcare services that are not considered essential health benefits.
    D. Yes, except for all hospitalizations.

56. **All medications had to be prescribed by a licensed practitioner before 1938.**

    A. True

    B. False

57. **Cash flow is the accounting term that describes**

    A. When you receive reimbursement.

    B. When you submit a claim.

    C. When you pay bills.

    D. When you receive money and when you spend money.

58. **What is a 276 message?**

    A. A denial

    B. A response

    C. An approval

    D. An inquiry

59. **Why are practitioners concerned about medical coding and billing errors?**

    A. Errors can be corrected and the revenue stream restored.

    B. Errors increase claim processing.

    C. Errors cause increase of revenue to the practice. Any increase of revenue has nearly the same effect as a patient who is bleeding. As the stream slows, the medical practice or healthcare facility slowly dies.

    D. Errors cause disruption of revenue to the practice. Any disruption of revenue has nearly the same effect as a patient who is bleeding. As the stream slows, the medical practice or healthcare facility slowly dies.

60. **Nurses are members of the healthcare team who are licensed to observe, assess, and record a patient's symptoms.**

    A. True

    B. False

61. **A physician can be held liable for his or her employee's actions because an agency exists.**

    A. True

    B. False

62. **A condition is**

    A. A group of practitioners in which the insurer will reimburse the insured if the practitioner cares for the insured.

    B. A set of circumstances in which the insurer will not reimburse the insured if an inclusion occurs.

C. A set of circumstances in which the insurer will reimburse the insured if an inclusion occurs.

D. A set of circumstances in which the insurer will reimburse the insured if an exclusion occurs.

63. Down code reimbursement is when the examiner lowers the reimbursement or changes the code to a lower cost procedures rather than denying the claim.

A. True

B. False

64. Employment prospects for medical insurance specialists will remain favorable because

A. Medical billing is becoming less important to the healthcare industry.

B. Medical billing is automated.

C. The changing landscape of the insurance industry ensures a demand for professionals well versed in navigating the new requirements.

D. Automated has eliminated all errors.

65. All medical coding and billing errors can be eliminated.

A. True

B. False

66. Speak in clear, pleasant tones to convey self-assurance when answering the telephone.

A. True

B. False

67. Case law is a rule created by a court when interpreting statutory law and administrative law.

A. True

B. False

68. A contract can be

A. Written

B. Verbal

C. Created by the actions of two people

D. All of the above

69. A healthcare provider who performs a totally wrongful and unlawful act commits

A. Misfeasance

B. Malfeasance

C. Nonfeasance

D. None of the above

70. **Blue Cross**

    A. Provides surgery coverage

    B. Provides prescription medical coverage

    C. Provides physician medical coverage

    D. Provides hospital medical coverage

71. **Indemnity healthcare plans focus on treating current illnesses.**

    A. True

    B. False

72. **Besides affecting a practice cash flows and patient relations, what else can happen when medical billing and coding errors occur?**

    A. The practitioner may lose respect from colleagues.

    B. The practitioner may be dropped by the insurer.

    C. The patient may be dropped by the insurer.

    D. Medical billing and coding errors can lead to an investigation by regulators or law enforcement agencies. An innocent mistake might be taken as evidence of possible fraud.

73. **You should target your resume to a specific employment opportunity.**

    A. True

    B. False

74. **The focus of managed-care plans is on maintaining good health and lowering the risk of developing more severe illness.**

    A. True

    B. False

75. **The promise to do something for consideration in a contract is called an** *offer*.

    A. True

    B. False

76. **The Social Security Act of 1965 created Medicare and Medicaid.**

    A. True

    B. False

77. **When a caller's request cannot be addressed immediately, detailed information about the request is written as part of a message given to the person who will respond to the call.**

    A. True

    B. False

78. **A revenue stream is**

    A. A product or service that is bought to bring in revenue.
    B. A product or service that is sold to bring in revenue.
    C. A product or service that is sold to pay premiums.
    D. None of the above.

79. **What is the easiest way to gather a patient's health insurance information?**

    A. Ask the patient to tell you the information.
    B. Ask the patient to complete an insurance information form.
    C. Make a copy of the patient's health insurance card.
    D. Call the patient's health insurer.

80. **What should you be able to do within 10 seconds of reading your resume?**

    A. Tell if you are reliable.
    B. Tell if you are certified.
    C. Tell if you meet the job requirements.
    D. Tell if you are competent.

81. **The experienced rating system sets a premium based on the experience of the person who is being insured.**

    A. True
    B. False

82. **CBC is a test used during pregnancy to diagnose birth defects.**

    A. True
    B. False

83. **During the adjudication process, every aspect of the claim is examined and compared to terms of the group policy that covers the patient.**

    A. True
    B. False

84. **Miscoding a claim can get you sued as a vendor because the healthcare provider loses money because of your mistake.**

    A. True
    B. False

85. **Payment by an insurer to a healthcare provider for a claim is called a**

    A. Premium
    B. Reimbursement
    C. Differential
    D. Fee

86. **An angiography is a(n)**

    A. Sample of the amniotic fluid surrounding a fetus.

    B. X-ray scan used to measure the density of your bones.

    C. X-ray of blood vessels.

    D. X ray of arteries.

87. **An insurer should respond within 14 days from the date that the claim is filed. The medical insurance specialist should follow up with the insurer on the 15th day if there isn't a response to the claim.**

    A. True

    B. False

88. **Sick insurance was**

    A. An early version of medical insurance

    B. Similar to disability insurance

    C. Burial insurance

    D. All of the above

89. **A penalty can be applied if the healthcare provider violates a clause in an agreement with the insurer.**

    A. True

    B. False

90. **Why does a practitioner order medical tests?**

    A. To identify symptoms of a disease

    B. To gather additional objective information about the patient's conditions

    C. To increase reimbursements

    D. To reassure the patient about the prescribed treatment

91. **All contracts are voidable.**

    A. True

    B. False

92. **Health insurers are moving away from a fee-for-service model.**

    A. True

    B. False

93. **Patient information can be filed using the**

    A. Alphabetical filing system

    B. Numeric filing system

    C. Color-coding filing system

    D. All of the above

94. **Blue Cross and Blue Shield set policy rates using the community rating system.**

    A. True
    B. False

95. **A for-profit healthcare facility pays property taxes, income taxes, and sales tax.**

    A. True
    B. False

96. **Many medical insurance specialists attend a formal training program.**

    A. True
    B. False

97. **A healthcare provider who does not perform a lawful act when it should have been performed commits**

    A. Misfeasance
    B. Malfeasance
    C. Nonfeasance
    D. None of the above

98. **A colonoscopy is an examination of the inside of the colon.**

    A. True
    B. False

99. **The courts must create all terms of a contract.**

    A. True
    B. False

100. **A reason for implementing ICD-10-CM is the increase of the amount of available diagnosis to 68,000 possible diagnosis codes.**

    A. True
    B. False

Final Exam Answers

1. C. Recording of the brain's electrical activity.
2. C. A premium.
3. B. An encounter is whenever the patient engages the practitioner for service.
4. B. False.
5. C. Noncompliance.
6. B. The process of matching a claim on the remittance advice with claims submitted to the insurer.
7. B. Symptoms.
8. B. The insurer needs to be sure that claims received on behalf of his client are covered by the client's insurance policy before the healthcare provider is reimbursed.
9. B. False.
10. D. All of the above.
11. D. All of the above.
12. B. False.
13. B. Negligence.
14. B. Double booking.
15. A. Insuring a group of people.
16. A. The policy that is in effect the longest is the primary policy.
17. B. The patient may be charged amounts not reimbursed by the insurer as a result of medical billing and coding errors.
18. B. Healthcare providers who do not participate in the payer's program.
19. D. The capabilities of the body to repair itself.
20. A. Elderly and disabled who experience mounting medical bills.
21. D. All of the above.
22. A. Liver inflammation.

23. A. Licensed to perform some of a practitioner's duties under the direct supervision of a practitioner.
24. B. False.
25. D. Once verified, the claim is approved for payment and the healthcare provider is sent a remittance advice (RA) that details all the procedures that were listed on the claim and the reimbursement for each of them.
26. D. Double billing.
27. A. True.
28. A. True.
29. A. True.
30. A. True.
31. B. You first must estimate your healthcare expenses without medical coverage.
32. B. False.
33. B. False.
34. A. Gingivitis.
35. A. True.
36. C. Medical records specialist.
37. C. Use the medical insurer's Web site, by telephone, or through an insurance eligibility verification system.
38. A. True.
39. A. True.
40. B. False.
41. A. True.
42. B. False.
43. C. Transfer of reimbursements directly into the healthcare provider's bank account.
44. B. False.
45. A. True.
46. A. Computerized image of the metabolic activity of body tissues.
47. A. True.
48. A. True.
49. A. True.
50. A. True.
51. A. The Joint Commission accredits hospitals and establishes standards for healthcare facilities.
52. A. True.
53. A. Sent by the insurer to the patient when the claim is adjudicated.
54. A. True.
55. C. Yes, however, lifetime limits can apply to healthcare services that are not considered essential health benefits.
56. B. False.
57. D. When you receive money and when you spend money.
58. D. An inquiry.

59. D. Errors cause disruption of revenue to the practice. Any disruption of revenue has nearly the same effect as a patient who is bleeding. As the stream slows, the medical practice or healthcare facility slowly dies.

60. A. True.

61. A. True.

62. C. A set of circumstances in which the insurer will reimburse the insured if an inclusion occurs.

63. A. True.

64. C. The changing landscape of the insurance industry ensures a demand for professionals well versed in navigating the new requirements.

65. B. False.

66. A. True.

67. A. True.

68. D. All of the above.

69. D. None of the above.

70. D. Provides hospital medical coverage.

71. A. True.

72. D. Medical billing and coding errors can lead to an investigation by regulators or law enforcement agencies. An innocent mistake might be taken as evidence of possible fraud.

73. A. True.

74. A. True.

75. A. True.

76. A. True.

77. A. True.

78. B. A product or service that is sold to bring in revenue.

79. C. Make a copy of the patient's health insurance card.

80. C. Tell if you meet the job requirements.

81. A. True.

82. B. False.

83. A. True.

84. A. True.

85. B. Reimbursement.

86. C. X-ray of blood vessels.

87. A. True.

88. B. Similar to disability insurance.

89. A. True.

90. B. To gather additional objective information about the patient's conditions.

91. B. False.

92. A. True.

93. D. All of the above.

94. A. True.

95. A. True.
96. A. True.
97. B. Malfeasance.
98. A. True.
99. B. False.
100. A. True.

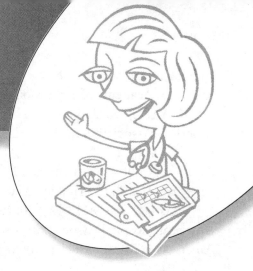

Index

Note: Page numbers followed by "*t*" refer to content found in table.